A Comprehensive and Practical Guide to Clinical Trials

A Comprehensive and Practical Guide to Clinical Trials

Edited by

Delva Shamley
Brenda Wright

The Clinical Research Centre at the University of Cape Town,
Cape Town, Western Cape Province, South Africa

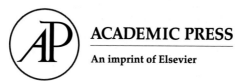

ACADEMIC PRESS

An imprint of Elsevier

Academic Press is an imprint of Elsevier
125 London Wall, London EC2Y 5AS, United Kingdom
525 B Street, Suite 1800, San Diego, CA 92101-4495, United States
50 Hampshire Street, 5th Floor, Cambridge, MA 02139, United States
The Boulevard, Langford Lane, Kidlington, Oxford OX5 1GB, United Kingdom

Notices
Knowledge and best practice in this field are constantly changing. As new research and experience broaden
our understanding, changes in research methods, professional practices, or medical treatment may become
necessary.

Practitioners and researchers must always rely on their own experience and knowledge in evaluating and
using any information, methods, compounds, or experiments described herein. In using such information or
methods they should be mindful of their own safety and the safety of others, including parties for whom they
have a professional responsibility.

To the fullest extent of the law, neither the Publisher nor the authors, contributors, or editors, assume any
liability for any injury and/or damage to persons or property as a matter of products liability, negligence or
otherwise, or from any use or operation of any methods, products, instructions, or ideas contained in the
material herein.

British Library Cataloguing-in-Publication Data
A catalogue record for this book is available from the British Library

Library of Congress Cataloging-in-Publication Data
A catalog record for this book is available from the Library of Congress

ISBN: 978-0-12-804729-3

For Information on all Academic Press publications
visit our website at https://www.elsevier.com/books-and-journals

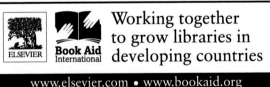

Working together
to grow libraries in
developing countries

www.elsevier.com • www.bookaid.org

Publisher: Mica Haley
Acquisition Editor: Kristine Jones and Erin Hill-Parks
Editorial Project Manager: Molly McLaughlin and Timothy Bennett
Production Project Manager: Lucía Pérez
Cover Designer: Matthew Limbert

Typeset by MPS Limited, Chennai, India

Contents

10. Data Management
Annemie Stewart

11. Investigational Medicinal Product (IMP) Management
Wynand Smythe and Nicky Kramer

List of Contributors

Nicky Kramer Clinical Research Centre, University of Cape Town, Cape Town, Western Cape Province, South Africa

Wynand Smythe Clinical Research Centre, University of Cape Town, Cape Town, Western Cape Province, South Africa

Annemie Stewart Clinical Research Centre, University of Cape Town, Cape Town, Western Cape Province, South Africa

Inge Vermeulen Clinical Research Centre, University of Cape Town, Cape Town, Western Cape Province, South Africa

Brenda Wright Clinical Research Centre, University of Cape Town, Cape Town, Western Cape Province, South Africa

Foreword

All research involving human participants, personal information, or biological samples must comply with adequate ethical and methodological standards. The need for providing public assurance that the rights, safety, and well-being of research participants are protected, and that data generated are credible, has been widely acknowledged at least since 1964, when the Declaration of Helsinki on the Ethical Principles for Medical Research Involving Human Subjects was first published. The importance of such public accountability will only keep on growing in today's context of "globalization of clinical trials," where medical research is carried out by commercial and noncommercial actors in a variety of settings in high-, middle-, and low-income countries, with increasingly complex challenges arising particularly in international collaborative research. These challenges include, for example, the need to engage with the research communities, while fairly sharing the research burdens and benefits; the difficulties to define adequate governance frames for data sharing and for research biobanks; and the exceptional challenges faced when research is carried out in the context of a public health emergency, as witnessed during the recent Ebola and Zika outbreaks.

In such an increasingly complex research environment, skilled and experienced clinicians and scientists are essential to build an efficient research site, but they are not enough. Clinical research teams also need to rely on adequate guidance and expertise in domains that go beyond medical and scientific skills. In the first place, they have to master the Good Clinical Practices (GCP) guidelines, which set the international standards for clinical research. In addition, in a competitive environment where medical research is often funded by external donors, they must be able to adequately and timely deal with contractual and administrative issues, as well as to ensure efficient planning and project management.

This book, grounded in the experience of a research group based in the South and fed by the experience of international collaborative research, timely addresses these needs. It provides a user-friendly guide to the different aspects of set-up and management of clinical research. Each chapter is integrated by a set of GCP-compliant forms and templates that may either be used as such, or adapted to the specificities of each study. It will provide an important support to research teams for building and consolidating local research capacity and for successfully conducting individual studies, either clinical trials with investigational medicinal products or other medical research studies. In addition, while the core-package of essential skills and standards tools becomes available and functional, the investigators will also gain the capacity and time to contextualize standard tools, to develop innovative approaches to newly emerging challenges, and to ensure research preparedness for outbreaks or other emergencies.

Raffaella Ravinetto
Department of Public Health
Institute of Tropical Medicine
Antwerp, Belgium

Chapter 1

Introduction to Clinical Trials

Brenda Wright

Chapter Outline

The purpose of this book is to illustrate and provide guidelines and information for planning and conducting a successful Clinical Trial from the Project Management perspective. Project Management is the application of planning, knowledge, skills, and technique to execute projects effectively and efficiently.

It will also describe the processes from beginning to end, and link these processes to key stakeholders and Good Clinical Practice (GCP), all of which are critical to the success of a trial (Table 1.1 and Fig. 1.1).

WHAT IS A CLINICAL TRIAL?

A Clinical Trial is a prospective biomedical or behavioral research project that involves human volunteers (participants) and/or uses materials of human origin, for example, observed behavior, answers to questions, and/or obtaining tissue or specimen samples.

WHY DO WE DO CLINICAL TRIALS?

Clinical trials are designed to answer a specific research question. They are used to determine if a new biomedical or behavioral intervention is safe, efficacious, and effective.

A Comprehensive and Practical Guide to Clinical Trials.
DOI: http://dx.doi.org/10.1016/B978-0-12-804729-3.00001-8

TABLE 1.1 What Is Good Clinical Practice?

GCP provides guidelines as defined by the ICH, an international body which defines standards that governments can transpose into regulations for clinical trials involving humans. These standards are referred to as ICH-GCP or ISO-GCP.

It is a standard for clinical trials, which includes the design, conduct, performance, monitoring, termination, auditing, recording, analysis, reporting, and documentation of clinical trials. These standards ensure that the trials are scientifically and ethically sound and that the clinical properties of the pharmaceutical product under investigation are properly documented and the data and reported results are credible and accurate. It also ensures that the rights, integrity, and confidentiality of trial participants are protected.

GCP guidelines therefore protect the human rights of participants in a clinical trial and provide assurance of the safety and efficacy of the newly developed compound. These guidelines also require detailed documentation for the clinical protocol, record keeping, training, and facilities, including computers and software. It defines the roles and responsibilities of clinical trial sponsors, clinical research investigators, and monitors. Quality assurance and inspections ensure that these standards are met.

The aim of GCP is to provide Investigators and their study teams with the tools to protect human subjects and collect quality data.

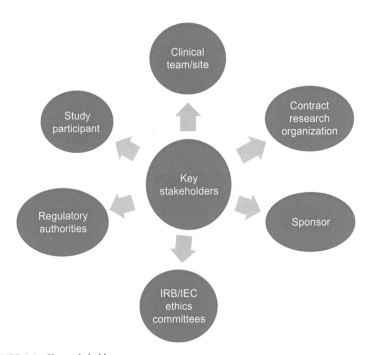

FIGURE 1.1 Key stakeholders.

Good Research Questions are:

- *Clear*. They are easy to understand and unambiguous.
- *Specific*. They are specific enough to understand what constitutes an answer.
- *Answerable*. It is clear what data we need, to answer the questions, and how the data will be collected.
- *Interconnected*. All the questions are related in some meaningful way, forming a coherent whole.
- *Substantively relevant*. They are nontrivial questions that are fundamentally worthy of the research effort and cost.

Some approaches are:

- To evaluate interventions (drugs, medical devices, etc.) for treating a disease, syndrome, or condition.
- To evaluate interventions that will identify or diagnose a particular disease or condition.
- To find methods to prevent the onset or recurrence of a disease or condition (medicine, vaccines, lifestyle changes, etc.).
- To investigate and identify methods to improve quality of life and comfort for patients with chronic illnesses.

These approaches have to follow GCP guidelines as defined by the International Council for Harmonization (ICH) and subsequently adapted in many countries (Table 1.1).

CLINICAL TEAM

The Sponsor or its contracted research organization (CRO) will appoint an Investigator Site consisting of the Principal Investigator and his/her Clinical Team who will conduct the clinical trial. In many countries the research team will be provided by a Clinical Trials Unit (CTU), which is based within the institution. On others, a CRO may provide all the research staff.

STUDY PARTICIPANT

A voluntary, informed person who has read and signed the Informed Consent Document, agreeing to the procedures, etc. he/she will be involved in during a Clinical Trial.

MEDICINES REGULATORY AUTHORITIES

In the case of trials involving an investigative medicinal product, regulatory requirements include approval by a medicines regulatory authority (MRA). The MRA is responsible for ensuring that all clinical trials of both nonregistered medicines, and new indications of registered medicines, comply with the necessary requirements for safety, quality, and efficacy. Applications for clinical trials and for registration of medicines and medical devices are reviewed by a MRA expert committee, which considers among other issues the scientific, medical, and ethical issues of the applications. Reports on the progress of the study are sent to the MRA on a regular basis. Proof of safety, quality, and efficacy must be submitted when applying to the Medicines Control Council (MCC) for approval and registration of a medicine for use in South Africa.

In the United States the regulatory body is the FDA (Food and Drug Administration) and in Europe it is the EMEA (European Agency for the Evaluation of Medicinal Products). In South Africa the MCC is the statutory body that regulates the performance of clinical trials and registration of medicines and medical devices for use in specific diseases. See Chapter 4, Regulatory Requirements, for more detailed information regarding International Regulatory submissions.

IRB/IEC ETHICS COMMITTEES

Approval by an institutional review board (IRB), or ethics board, is necessary prior to the conduct of a clinical trial. The IRB should consist of clinicians, researchers, and members from the community. They play an important role in ensuring that the trial is ethical, and that the welfare and human rights of the participants are protected according to GCP guidelines and the protection of personal information. The IRB inspects the trial for medical safety and protection of the participants involved in the trial, prior to approval.

SPONSOR

The Sponsor can be an individual, company, institution, or organization that has the responsibility to initiate and manage the clinical trial. The sponsor may or may not provide the funding. It may be a governmental organization, a pharmaceutical, and biotechnology or medical device company. The clinical trial may also be managed by an outsourced partner, i.e., a contract research organization (CRO) or an academic clinical trial unit. National health agencies and academic institutions may offer grants to Investigators who design clinical trials that attempt to answer research questions of interest to the agency or institution. A study initiated by an investigator from academia is known as an Investigator Lead Trial (ILT) and usually the academic institution acts as the regulatory sponsor.

CONTRACT RESEARCH ORGANIZATIONS

A CRO provides support to the pharmaceutical, biotechnology, and medical device industries in performing one or more of the trial-related duties and functions, i.e., to conduct clinical research trials on behalf of the Sponsor. The CRO is contracted by a pharmaceutical, medical device, or biotechnology company (Sponsor). CROs employ various clinical research associates, biostatisticians, medical writers, project managers, and similar clinical research professionals to support the conduct of clinical trials on behalf of their pharmaceutical, biotech, and medical device company sponsors. A CRO will also review and validate (monitor) the trial data during the clinical trial. Other CRO services may include medical writing, regulatory support, investigator/site selection and qualification, clinical trial management, and data analysis (biostatistics). CROs are not routinely used in ILTs.

MANAGING THE TRIAL

Management of the trial process requires a fluidity of steps summarized in Figs. 1.2−1.4 and illustrates the systematic approach to be followed in order to successfully conduct a clinical trial. During this time, the stakeholders each has their specific roles to play and certain steps must be in place before continuing with the next.

There are three stages to the process, each of which is described below:

Section 1 illustrates the first stage and discusses the development of the study drug, the research question, and the regulatory requirements.

Some of these processes may happen simultaneously and not necessarily in the exact order as illustrated below, but they all have to be in place before the conduct of a clinical trial can commence.

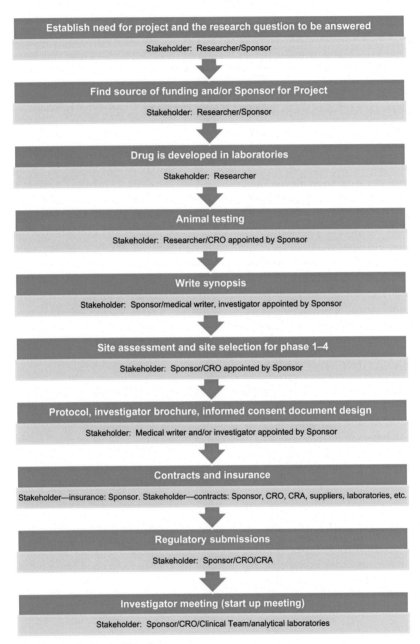

FIGURE 1.2 Section 1—Flowchart.

Section 2 illustrates the planning and training stage.

During this time, the clinical team will plan the conduct and make sure that all documents, contracts, supplies are in place. Training of staff is done and specific duties are allocated by the principal investigator. This stage of a clinical trial sometimes may take longer than conducting the actual trial. However, meticulous planning is essential for success.

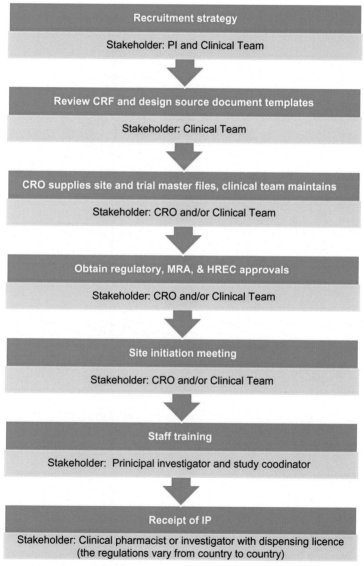

FIGURE 1.3   Section 2—Flowchart.

Section 3 illustrates the conduct of the clinical trial and what happens when a trial closes.

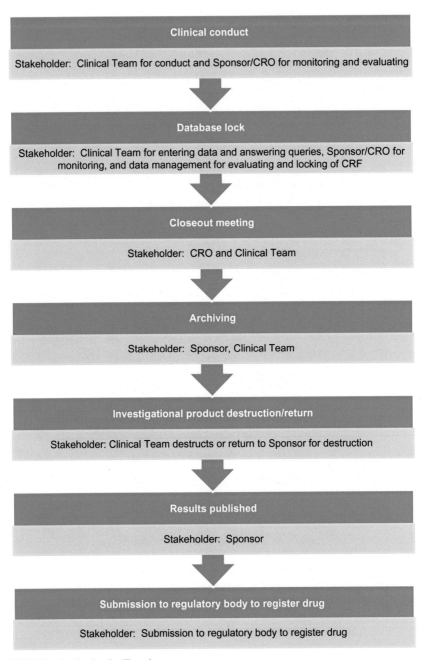

FIGURE 1.4   Section 3—Flowchart.

Keypoints
- Research Question—Clinical trials are designed to answer a specific Research question. It defines the study design and outcomes to be met.
- GCP—Good clinical practice should be followed throughout the research project.
- Key Stakeholders—Know who they are and where they fit into the trial.
- Process Flow—Strategic planning will ensure the systematic flow of your project from beginning to end.

FURTHER READING

ICH Harmonised Tripartite Guideline E6 (R1), Current step 4 version dated 10 June 1996.
https://clinicaltrials.gov/ct2/about-studies/learn.
https://grants.nih.gov/grants/funding/phs398/instructions2/p2_human_subjects_definitions.htm.
U.S. Department of Health and Human Services/Clinical Research Definitions and Procedures.
SNM Clinical Trials Network.

Chapter 2

Clinical Trial Phases

Chapter Outline

As illustrated in Chapter 1, Introduction to Clinical Trials, before the conduct of clinical trials, research companies will have conducted extensive preclinical studies (laboratory and animal studies) for activity and toxicity data. Once it has passed through these tests, studies of safety and toxicity may be conducted in human volunteers, with careful clinical monitoring. A series of clinical studies with increasing number of participants must be conducted before a new product can be introduced for widespread use.

Clinical trials involving new drugs are conducted in a series of sequential steps called phases to determine the safety and tolerability of the new drug and the efficacy against the target disease(s).

Each phase is designed to answer a separate research question and is a separate clinical trial. Clinical trials are generally classified into Phases I to IV. It is not possible to draw distinct lines between the phases, and diverging opinions about definitions and methodology do exist. An investigational product can be evaluated in more than one phase simultaneously in different clinical trials, and some clinical trials may overlap two different phases.

In this chapter we look at the different Clinical Trial Phases and the key aims of each phase as this defines the scope of work and thus the project managers' responsibilities.

A Comprehensive and Practical Guide to Clinical Trials.
DOI: http://dx.doi.org/10.1016/B978-0-12-804729-3.00002-X
11

PHASE I

Phase I studies are exploratory first-into-human or early phase trials, designed to make an assessment of the safety and tolerability of a new drug or vaccine in a small group of people (usually healthy volunteers, but in some therapeutic areas, like cancer, the participants are patients) as well as to determine the maximum tolerated dose (MTD).

The new study drug is administered in small doses at first and then ascended to larger doses to gather preliminary data on the pharmacokinetic (the concentration of the new drug and its metabolites and where it is absorbed) and pharmacodynamic (what the new drug does in the body) effects.

Phase I trials help to determine the correct dose and frequency that are safe and necessary to have an effect.

In this phase (and indeed all phases), it is critical to monitor, identify, and report all side effects (Adverse Events).

PROOF-OF-CONCEPT TRIALS

These trials are conducted at an early stage of clinical drug development. This step of proof-of-concept often links Phase I and dose ranging Phase II trials. The trials are conducted on a small-scale and are normally designed to estimate whether one compound might have clinically significant efficacy in other diseases, besides the disease for which it was originally developed, or is further development warranted. From medicines regulatory authority (MRA) perspective, this is known as a "new indication."

PHASE IIa AND PHASE IIb

In the absence of any safety concerns, the trial can move into Phase II.

The new drug is now tested on a larger number of participants and the protocol is designed to assess the effectiveness of the drug. The aim is to assess the activity, feasibility, and toxicity of a given dose.

Therapeutic drugs are tested on patients and vaccines in healthy participants to assess immunogenicity.

Safety evaluations are continued and intervals between doses may continue to be determined.

The new study drug may be tested in a number of Phase II trials, evaluating its performance under different circumstances, for example, initially tested in adults, but then tested in younger groups until tested in the final target population of infants.

Phase IIa

- All safety assessments compiled during Phase I can now be repeated on a much larger participant group.
- Phase IIa trials are pilot clinical trials that also evaluate efficacy in selected populations of patients with the disease or condition to be treated, diagnosed, or prevented.
- Objectives focus on dose requirements, that is, what is the MTD that is safe for participants to take, dose-response, type of patients, frequency of dosing, or numerous other characteristics of safety and efficacy.

Phase IIb

- Phase IIb trials focus on how well the drug works at the prescribed dose.
- They usually represent the most rigorous demonstration of a medicine's efficacy.
- Phase IIb trials are sometimes referred to as pivotal trials.
- A *pivotal trial* is intended to provide evidence for a drug-marketing approval. Phase III trials are assumed to be pivotal so the phrase is often used for the rare pivotal phase II trials.

Phase II trials will move onto the Phase III stage once it has been adequately demonstrated that the study drug is effective against the disease for which it is being tested.

PHASE IIIa AND PHASE IIIb

Phase III trials aim to provide a definitive assessment of the efficacy of the drug against the primary outcome(s) as well as providing safety data in a large group of participants.

The drug or treatment is given to even larger groups of people (1000−3000 or more) to confirm its effectiveness, monitor side effects, compare it to commonly used treatments, and collect information that will allow the drug or treatment to be used safely. The pattern and profile of frequent adverse events are investigated and special features of the drug are investigated.

These trials should preferably be of a randomized double blind design, but other designs are acceptable (e.g., long-term safety trials).

They are often referred to as "*pivotal trials*" as they are conducted to produce the evidence of efficacy and safety required to submit a new drug to a licensing authority.

Phase IIIa

- These trials are conducted after efficacy of the study drug is demonstrated but before the submission of a New Drug Application.
- They are conducted in patient populations for which the medicine is intended.
- Additional data are generated on safety and efficacy in large numbers of patients.
- They often provide much of the information needed for the package insert and labeling of the medicine.

Phase IIIb

- Phase IIIb trials are conducted after the regulatory submission of a New Drug Application, but before the medicine's approval and marketing.
- This phase accumulates additional findings and information which may be required by the regulatory authority prior to approval.
- These trials supplement earlier trials, complete earlier trials, or may be directed toward new types of trials or Phase IV trials.

PHASE IV

Phase IV trials are done after the drug or treatment has been marketed to gather information on the drug's effect in various populations and any side effects associated with long-term use.

They are usually postregistration or postlicensure trials and provide additional details about the medicine's long-term efficacy or safety profiles.

These trials are conducted to assess the effectiveness of a new drug when it is used in a public environment, as compared to the efficacy assessed in a carefully controlled Phase III trial.

New age groups, populations, and other medicine comparisons can be evaluated.

Important safety issues that only arise in a relatively small proportion of people may only be reported during this phase due to the widespread use of the new drug.

These trials should use the same scientific and ethical standards as applied in premarketing studies.

Keypoints

Phase I	Exploratory first-into-human or early phase
	Pharmacokinetic and pharmacodynamic effects, and MTD
Proof of concept	Determines clinical significance in other diseases
	Is further development warranted?
Phase II	Initial investigation of treatment activity (assess effectiveness of drug)
	Larger number of participants
	Determine correct doses and intervals between doses
Phase III	Full-scale comparative treatment evaluation
	Produce evidence of efficacy and safety required for submission to licensing authority
Phase IV	Postmarketing surveillance
	Assess effectiveness in public environment
	New age groups, populations, and comparisons can be evaluated
	Widespread use may detect important safety issues that only arise in small proportion of people

FURTHER READING

medical-dictionary.the free dictionary.com/Phase + 3b" > /a > accessed on 22 February 2016
http://www.nlm.nih.gov/services/ctphases.html.

Chapter 3

Setting Up of Site, Site Assessment Visits, and Selection

Brenda Wright

Chapter Outline

Now that we understand the different phases of clinical trials as discussed in Chapter 2, Clinical Trial Phases, we can ensure that our trial facility fits the requirements necessary for the phases and therapeutic areas we will concentrate on.

Participant data gathered through the process of Research and Development and performed by a network of clinical sites and study centers are the backbone of drug development. Pharmaceutical companies devote billions of dollars into a cycle of bench, laboratory, animal, and finally human research. According to Good Clinical Practice (GCP), it is the responsibility of the Sponsor Company to choose a site that is qualified to conduct research, has proper training, and has adequate resources to successfully conduct a clinical trial. The Investigator Site should demonstrate the potential and time for recruiting required number of suitable subjects within the agreed recruitment period. The Investigator should have adequate, qualified staff, and facilities for the duration of the trial (see Sections 4.2.3, 5.6.1, and 5.18.4). The International Council for Harmonization (ICH) guidelines give Sponsors and CROs sufficient room to apply their subsets of criteria in the selection process. Their criteria are more or less projected in the standard operating procedures (SOPs) of the company or institution that performs the investigator site selection.

A Comprehensive and Practical Guide to Clinical Trials.
DOI: http://dx.doi.org/10.1016/B978-0-12-804729-3.00003-1

In order to meet all the requirements of sample size and demographics, and conduct the research in a timely manner, many investigator sites may be required worldwide. This constitutes an enormous investment in both money and time for the Sponsor. There are various costs involved in setting up a site that complies with all these requirements. Some of these costs include training site personnel on protocol-specific requirements, GCP requirements, Institutional Review Board (IRB) reporting requirements, the use of outside contractors for equipment and consumables. There are also traveling costs, initiation, monitoring, close-out visits, and ongoing patient recruitment and retention costs. Other costs involve staff time worked and site management.

SETTING UP OF SITE

Industry sponsors will conduct a feasibility study first, followed by a visit to the site where the trial will be conducted to determine if the potential site meets all the study requirements. They would look at not only the functionality of the site for research purposes, but also it meets the basic requirements for most clinical trials as described below. The Sponsor's marketing department and/or the CRO Company will decide on which countries to choose and how many sites in each country will be used. The CRO will appoint a monitor to collect information about the potential sites. All details regarding the potential sites are then presented to the Sponsor with recommendations and the Sponsor makes the final decision of which sites to use.

In setting up a clinical trial site, the following basic requirements are necessary:

- *General Requirements*

  Make sure that the area where participants are seen and where research activities will take place is clean and well organized. The waiting area should be comfortable and well lit.
- *Drug/Investigational Product (IMP)/Pharmacy Room*

  It is the responsibility of the site to take the appropriate measures to ensure IMP security.

  IMP should be kept in a secure (limited access), temperature controlled, and locked room. If more than one study is conducted at the site concurrently, investigational product (IP) should be kept in separate locked cabinets in the IP room, clearly marked with Protocol Numbers. Sponsor names and IP codes/names should not be on display. Locked cabinets also minimize clutter and the collection of dust. Sites must be able to provide proof of continuous temperature monitoring as well as back-up plans in the case of electricity failure and/or air conditioning malfunction.

  All equipment used in the IP room must be appropriately calibrated as per manufacturer's specifications and proof of calibration must be available.

Chapter 12, Collecting, Processing, and Shipment of Blood and Urine Samples, describes pharmacy-related requirements in further detail.

- *Examination Rooms/Admission Wards*

  These rooms must comply with local and state requirements including OSHA (Occupational Safety & Health Act). Rooms should be spacious and well lit. For Phase 1 trials, access, including windows, must be secured and controlled. Medical emergency procedures should be well documented (SOP) and tested. Emergency trolleys/crash carts must comply with regulatory requirements and maintained on a regular basis.

- *Process Laboratory/Transit Laboratory*

  If sites process samples for shipment, this should be done in a temperature controlled room. Processed samples stored in fridges and freezers must be in a room with secure access. As with the pharmacy, sites must be able to provide proof of continuous temperature monitoring as well as back-up plans in the case of electricity failure and/or air conditioning malfunction. In the case of a power failure or freezer error, a system must be in place to alert key staff via phone messages.

  All equipment used in the laboratory room must be appropriately calibrated as per manufacturer's specifications. Proof of regular calibration must be available.

  Staff responsible for preparing dangerous goods for shipment (e.g., dry ice shipments) must have IATA (International Air Transport Association) or other equivalent international certification.

- *Storage Areas*

  Fire proof lockable filing cabinets should be available to store study documents (site files, source documents, supplies, etc.). These should be clearly marked with the Protocol Number, but not Sponsor name and/or IP codes.

  Long-term storage of study documents (archiving) should be arranged if not available on the premises and should comply with all regulations.

- *Work Area for Study Coordinator, Data Capturers, and Monitor*

The study coordinator and data capturer (if applicable) will need a dedicated work area to complete administration duties. They will need data ports and desktop computers/laptops for planning, communication, and electronic data entry duties. Sometimes sponsor-specific hardware and software will be used and so enough space must be created to accommodate the equipment. Site computers with participant/patient data should be secure and password protected.

Some trials may require frequent on-site visits by the sponsor's or CRO's monitor. They will require a quiet location where confidentiality is not compromised. Desk space should be large enough to accommodate multiple open files and case report books and/or laptops where applicable. Telephone, copier, and fax machine access is optional but beneficial.

FEASIBILITY

Once you have ticked all the boxes as described above, you are ready to look at feasibilities and prepare for your site assessment visits.

Feasibility is one of the first steps taken in clinical trials and focusses on patient availability and the potential to meet the recruitment target. During this process, your site gets an opportunity to review a clinical trial synopsis and/or protocol to assess whether the study is a good fit for your site.

The CRO/Sponsor Company will contact the Principal Investigator or Site director to discuss a proposed clinical trial. A nondisclosure agreement is signed where necessary by the site and returned, prior to the feasibility documents being forwarded to the site. You will then use these documents, usually a protocol synopsis and questionnaire, to assess the suitability for your site.

Depending on the information available, you could perform a provisional Risk Assessment during this time as well (see Chapter 15, Quality Management, for more information on Risk Assessment), but the outcome of the Risk Assessment is not necessarily the deciding factor. For example, a high-risk trial (first into human, etc.) should not be refused if the site is capable of conducting such a trial.

There is no valid reason to say no to a trial during the feasibility stage unless it is professionally or ethically unacceptable or the patient base is not available.

SITE ASSESSMENT VISITS

Site Selection Criteria

- A proactive systematic plan is key to successfully selecting the appropriate sites.
- Selectors must determine how many sites to select and where they should be geographically.
- In order to find potential investigators, selectors will define qualifications necessary for given trial.
- They will match the potential site characteristics to the specific needs of the study.
- There are certain critical success factors to selecting the optimal site to conduct a Clinical Trial, that is, what constitutes an ideal site?
  - With the increasing complexity of study protocols and regulatory requirements, the Sponsor's main focus is ensuring that the site they choose employs trained and experienced staff (especially the PI and study coordinator) who understand the complexities and pitfalls of conducting clinical research.
  - Recruitment and enrollment capabilities and strength of patient database.

- IRB and regulatory timelines. Potential country-specific timelines and special requirements will be a deciding factor. Countries where the submission to approval time is short will be more likely to be selected as a suitable geographical area to select sites.
- Secured drug storage area with the necessary temperature controls in place.
- Site's ability to perform specialized trial procedures, blood collection, processing, and shipping of samples.
- Selectors will look at possible competing trials that may interfere with their project.
- Experience in conducting trials involving Electronic Data Capturing and interactive Web response systems.
- An important factor will be the influence of the PI in the industry (i.e., Key Opinion Leader in the field), PI/site affiliation (either with a larger consortium or an academic institution), and whether the site or PI has had any regulatory audits, findings, warning letters, or violations.
- In addition to this, they need sufficient proof that the Investigator and the rest of the staff are available to conduct the trial and whether the sites' current workload is manageable.
- Estimated costs per completed participant in addition to other site costs associated with the trial.

Site Visits

During a Site Assessment visit, it is essential that key site personnel are available to discuss all information the Sponsor's representative may want to know. It is therefore necessary to set the visit date so that it suits all relevant staff members. Depending on the site set-up, the following staff members should always attend a site assessment meeting:

- Principal Investigator;
- Study Coordinator (in specialist trial sites with multiple coordinators, the coordinator may not have been identified for a specific trial at this stage. In this case the Project Manager/Clinical Operations Manager will represent the study coordinator);
- Project Manager/Clinical Operations Manager (ClinOps);
- Site Director (if applicable);
- Pharmacist (if applicable).

It is also beneficial to prepare for the site visit. It leaves a professional impression with the representative if documents and information normally required during site assessment visits are immediately available. For specialized trial sites with experience in more than one therapeutic area, a short presentation by the Site Director showing photos, metrics including number of studies conducted in various therapeutic areas (past, ongoing, and future), and enrollment rates and screen failure rates (based on sites' past experience in the particular therapeutic area) will be welcomed by the Sponsor representative and is a good marketing tool for future business. See Table 3.1 and Fig. 3.1 as an example. Offer the presentation (printed or on a flash-drive) to the representative to take away with them.

TABLE 3.1 History of Site's Clinical Trials

Phase I—First-Into-Man Trial

Objective	To evaluate the safety, tolerability, and pharmacokinetic properties of escalating single and multiple doses administered to healthy participants
Scope	• Single center • Ascending single and multiple dose • Eight participants per dose cohort
Challenge	• Strict Inclusion/Exclusion criteria • Short timelines • Data entry within 24 hours
Actions	• Ongoing proactive Recruitment • Used ACLS trained paramedics and nurses • Staff compliment increased as necessary to cope with increased workload • Ongoing training and feedback meetings after each admission period • Weekly status report sent to monitor and clinical team
Outcome	• 202 participants screened. 80% of screen failures due to safety blood results • 48 participants dosed • 48 participants completed • Trial finished after six cohorts due to variability in pharmacokinetics (PK) results

Phase II—Pediatric

Objective	To evaluate the safety, efficacy, and the relationship between study drug and the inhibition of platelet aggregation in pediatric patients, using PK-PD modeling
Scope	• Multicenter • Open-label followed by a double blind, placebo-controlled extension phase
Challenge	• Trial was conducted off-site. Space was limited and spread out • Difficult patient population • Strict Inclusion/Exclusion criteria • Rigorous PK and pharmacodynamics (PD) sampling on young children
Actions	• Lead Investigator checked database on a weekly basis to identify potential patients • Thorough prescreening was done and detailed discussions held with the parents and patients prior to screening

(Continued)

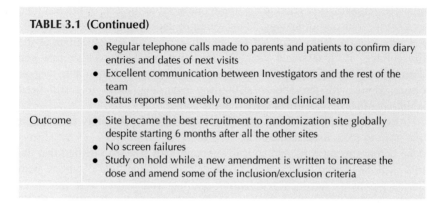

TABLE 3.1 (Continued)

	• Regular telephone calls made to parents and patients to confirm diary entries and dates of next visits • Excellent communication between Investigators and the rest of the team • Status reports sent weekly to monitor and clinical team
Outcome	• Site became the best recruitment to randomization site globally despite starting 6 months after all the other sites • No screen failures • Study on hold while a new amendment is written to increase the dose and amend some of the inclusion/exclusion criteria

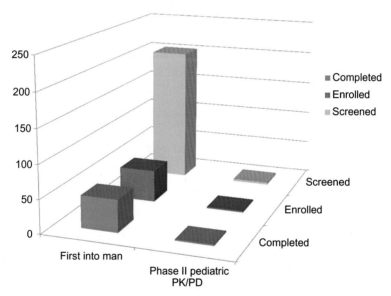

FIGURE 3.1   Graphic showing trial history at site.

A checklist (Appendix 3.1) can be used prior to the meeting to ensure that the site is prepared and have all the necessary documents/information at the ready when the Sponsor/monitor arrives. This checklist can be coordinated by the Project Manager or any other staff member depending on the set-up of the site. Responsible persons will also vary from site to site and country to country. This list is beneficial to keep as part of the metrics of your site and to keep your site data updated.

Questions to ask are not set in stone and each site should select their own. These questions are very dependent on the nature of the trial and the site requirements. It is good to ask these questions at the end of the meeting, as a lot of your questions may be answered by the representative during his/ her presentation. They may not be able to answer all the questions at the time of the site assessment visit, but it shows the representative that you are interested and proactive in what is expected of you. It may also trigger certain alerts with the Sponsor Company regarding issues that still need addressing that they may not have thought about.

Always remember that this visit is also the site's opportunity to assess if you want to participate in the conduct of the trial. Feasibilities are not always done before this meeting and so it is important that you are satisfied that the trial will be within your scope of practice and expertise, complies with Ethical standards and local regulations, and that you will be able to deliver quality data on time.

KEY QUESTIONS TO ASK

- What are the predicted timelines for the trial?
- Who will be doing the regulatory submissions? (In some countries the CRO or Site can be responsible for this.)
- How many sites if a multisite trial, will be participating, specifically how many in your country and/or city?
- How many participants will the site be responsible for enrolling and will it be competitive recruitment?
- How long will the recruitment period be and what is the recruitment/ enrollment ratio?
- Will you be using a central laboratory or local laboratories for safety tests?
- How will IP be stored? Room temperature, refrigerated?
- Which courier will be used for shipment of samples? (If the Sponsor is thinking of using a courier that your site has had a bad experience with, now is the time to notify them and inform them of the courier of choice in your city and/or country.) If the courier has not been decided yet, mention your preference and why.
- Will any specialist equipment be supplied by the Sponsor? (e.g., specific ECG instruments, infusion pumps, incubators, water baths, etc.)

Other factors to take into consideration would be the interests of the parties involved in the site selection process.

Sponsor/Marketing Department: They need a product of high quality with unique features to compete with the rest of the world. They also need to perform the trial as quickly as possible to shorten the time period to marketing.

Sponsor/Clinical Department: This department will have a set budget to work with. For them, it is vitally important that the trial is conducted in time, but that the data are of a high quality, thus limiting queries.

CRO: The CRO will spend little time on feasibility as it is typically unpaid work done. They have the same goals as the Clinical Department above.

Investigator Site: Not too much time can be spent on the decision as it is not time paid for. Sites have to deliver high-quality data on time as it is an important marketing tool for future business.

Keypoints

- According to GCP, it is the responsibility of the Sponsor Company to choose a site that is qualified to conduct research, has proper training, and has adequate resources to successfully conduct a clinical trial.
- The Investigator Site should demonstrate the potential and time for recruiting required number of suitable subjects within the agreed recruitment period.
- The Investigator should have adequate, qualified staff, and facilities for the duration of the trial.
- Sponsors would normally appoint a Clinical Research Organisation (CRO) to conduct an on-site qualification visit to determine if the potential site meets all the study requirements.
- During a Site Assessment visit, it is essential that key site personnel are available to discuss all information the Sponsor's representative may want to know.
- Use a checklist to help with the preparation of the site visit. This list can also be used for keeping site metrics.
- Be prepared to ask relevant questions regarding the trial.
- There is no valid reason to say no to a trial during the feasibility stage unless it is professionally or ethically unacceptable.

FURTHER READING

www.tklresearch.com/cra-services/.../feasibility-site.identification) accessed on 22 February 2016.

https://digital commons.hsc.unt.edu/cgi/viewcontent.cgi?article=1083 accessed on 22 February 2016.

APPENDIX 3.1 SITE ASSESSMENT VISIT CHECKLIST

Site Assessment Visit Checklist

	Date of Visit: _____
Therapeutic Area: _____	Principal Investigator: _____
Company Visiting: _____	Contact Name: _____

Item	Person Responsible	Comments	
Venue & Projector booked for meeting	Secretary		✓
Information provided by Sponsor, sent to all staff attending the meeting	Principal Investigator		✓
Meeting invite sent to all participating parties	Project Manager		✓
Notify Pharmacy and Lab personnel regarding the time of site tour	Project Manager		✓
Complete and sign all documents (if any) sent by Sponsor/Monitor prior to the meeting	Principal Investigator/ Project Manager		
Relevant SOPs available	Project Manager		
Calibration certificates available	Project Manager		
Temperature monitoring printouts available	Project Manager		
Emergency Trolley/crash cart with checklists ready for inspection	Study Coordinator/ ClinOps Manager		
Information regarding Regulatory and or Sponsor Audits	Project Manager	Have stats available regarding type of audits, dates, findings, and/or observations	
Organogram of Site Staff	Project Manager		
*Prepare specific questions to ask relevant to the proposed trial	All staff involved	Answers to be noted here	
Feedback from Company regarding selection	Principal Investigator/ Project Manager	Reason if not approved can be completed here	Yes/ No

Chapter 4

Regulatory Requirements

Inge Vermeulen

Chapter Outline

The regulatory requirements of a submission to conduct a clinical trial are dependent on the type of intervention. It is important to remember that not all clinical trials involve a novel drug. Clinical trials can also involve registered drugs that are being tested at a new dose, via a new route of administration or for a new indication. Furthermore, clinical trials can also investigate medical devices and/or new surgical interventions. These trials are often submitted to the national Medicine Regulatory Authorities (MRAs) in accordance with Investigational New Drug (IND) requirements; however, in many countries the regulation of clinical trials involving medical devices/surgical intervention is still underdeveloped. The focus of this chapter will remain on the submission requirements of Investigational New Drugs (INDs) specifically. Website URLs directing you to the MRA webpage will be provided in the reference list of this chapter for more information regarding the regulatory requirements and additional information for the submission of clinical trial application (CTA).

The regulatory requirements enforced by the country-specific national MRAs are governed by country-specific legislation, regulations, and guidelines. These legislations are binding to all parties whereas the regulations are instrumental to enforcing the legislation. Guidelines, such as International Council for Harmonization-Good Clinical Practice (ICH-GCP), highlight the standards of practice and although not legally binding, these guidelines are often referred to in the legislation and in this way enforced. The ICH-GCP guidelines were

A Comprehensive and Practical Guide to Clinical Trials.
DOI: http://dx.doi.org/10.1016/B978-0-12-804729-3.00004-3

unified in 1990 to protect the rights, safety, well-being of trial subjects, and to ensure the scientific integrity of data. These guidelines are now fundamental to the review and conduct of clinical trials. Institutional Review Boards (IRBs) [also known as Independent Ethics Committees (IEC) and/or Health Research Ethic Committees (HREC)] are representative of a nation or state and review CTAs in accordance with the Declaration of Helsinki (2013) and ICH-GCP. The MRAs serve as a national oversight for research involving human subjects and are responsible for the approval and registration of new medicines. The elected MRA committee will review the scientific, medical, and ethical aspects of an IND application and determine the impact it will have on public health in its respective country or state. The common technical document (CTD) standardizes the format of a submission by prompting the applicant to justify the submission with respect to the science, medical, and ethical aspects of the trial. The CTD is organized into five modules namely, administration, overall quality, quality data, nonclinical study reports, and clinical study reports (refer to Fig. 4.1). Although you can expect differences in the country-specific CTA submission processes and timelines, the following are prerequisites prior to enrollment of the first participant in any clinical trial involving an IND:

- approval from a national MRAs,
- approval from a registered IRB/HREC,
- registration with a National Clinical Registry accessible to the general public.

(The applicant should also confirm whether approval from the trial site, i.e., hospital or clinic is a necessary before participant enrollment.)

For the purpose of this chapter, we discuss the various regulatory bodies in more detail and how CTA requirements differ between countries, specifically in United States, Europe (member states), United Kingdom, South Africa, Australia, China, and India (Table 4.1).

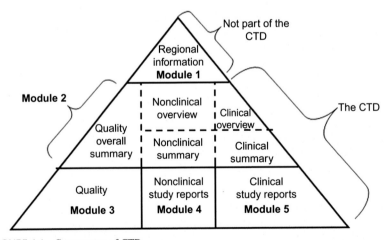

FIGURE 4.1   Components of CTD.

TABLE 4.1 The Legislation, Regulations, and Guidelines of the Country-Specific Regulatory Bodies for Research Involving Drugs and Devices

Country	National Regulatory Body	Legislation	Regulations	Guidelines
South Africa	Medicine Control Council (MCC)	Medicines and Related Substances Control Act, 101 of 1965	General Regulations Made in Terms of the Medicines and Related Substances Act, 1965 (2003) Ethics in Health Research Principles, Processes, and Structures (Second Edition, 2015)	Guidelines for Good Practice in the Conduct of Clinical Trials in Human Participants in South Africa (Second Edition, 2006)
	Department of Health (DoH)			
The United States	Food and Drug Administration (FDA)	Food, Drug, and Cosmetic Act, 21 USC Sections 355 and 371 (2012)	21 CFR parts; 50,312,56,314,807,812,814	General: GCP and Human Subject Protections in FDA-Regulated Clinical Trials
		Public Health Service Act, 42 USC Section 262 (1998)		
		FDA Administration Amendments Act 801		
		Food, Drug, and Cosmetic Act, 21 USC Section 360 (2012)		

(Continued)

TABLE 4.1 (Continued)

Country	National Regulatory Body	Legislation	Regulations	Guidelines
Europe	European Agency for the Evaluation of Medicinal Products (EMA) European Commission Member State Medicine Regulator	Directive 2001/20/EC (Clinical Trials Regulation EU No 536/2014)	Policy on Publication of Clinical Data for Medicinal Products for Human Use (2015)	Note for Guidance on GCP (CPMP/ICH/135/95) (1997)
		Directive 2001/83/EC		
		Directive 2005/28/EC		
		Regulation No. 536/2014		
		Directive 93/42/EEC		
		Directive 98/79/EC		
		Directive 2007/47/EC		
The United Kingdom	Medicines and Healthcare Products Regulatory Agency (MHRA)	Medicines Act (1968)		ICH-GCP
Australia	Therapeutic Goods Administration (TGA)	Therapeutic Goods Act 1989 (2015) National Health and Medical Research Council Act of (1992)	Therapeutic Goods Regulations 1990 (2015)	Human Research Ethics Committees and the Therapeutic Goods Administration (2001)
				Australian Clinical Trial Handbook (2006)
				Australian Regulatory Guidelines for Medical Devices (ARGMD)
				Good Clinical Research Practice (GCRP) Australia

Country	Agency	Law	Regulations	Guidelines
China	China Food and Drug Administration (CFDA)	Drug Administration Law of the People's Republic of China (2001)	Regulations for Implementation of the Drug Administration Law of the People's Republic of China (2002)	Guideline for HIV Vaccine Research Technology (2003)
			Chinese GCP (2003) (Mandarin)	Guideline for Vaccine Research Technology (2004)
			Special Review and Approval Procedure for Drug Registration of the State Food and Drug Administration (2005)	Guidelines on Ethical Review of Drug Clinical Trials (2010)
			Provisions for Drug Registration (2007)	
			Qualification and Evaluation of Clinical Trial Sites (2008)	
			Rules on the Administration of Report and Supervision of Adverse Drug Reactions (2010)	

(Continued)

TABLE 4.1 (Continued)

Country	National Regulatory Body	Legislation	Regulations	Guidelines
India	Central Drugs Standard Control Organization, Office of Drugs Controller General of India (DCGI)	Schedule Y of the Drugs and Cosmetics Act (2005)	GCPs for Clinical Research in India (2001)	Ethical Guidelines for Biomedical Research on Human Participants: Chapter IV. Drug Trials and Vaccine Trials (2006)
	Indian Council of Medical Research (ICMR)	Drugs & Cosmetics Act, 1940 (2005)	Permission for Clinical Trials: General Statutory Rules 63(E)	Ethical Guidelines for Biomedical Research on Human Participants: Clinical Trials with Surgical Procedures/Medical Devices
	Central Drugs Standard Control Organization (CDSCO)		Ethics Committee Registration: General Statutory Rules 72(E)	
	Indian Council of Medical Research (ICMR)		A/V Consent—General Statutory Rules 611 (E) (2015)	
			Rules: Schedule D & K	

IRB/IEC ETHICS COMMITTEES

In line with ICH-GCP guidelines, the IRB consists of physicians, researchers, and members from the community who review and evaluate the medical aspects and ethics of a proposed trial to safeguard the rights, safety, and well-being of all trial subjects, especially those considered to be of a vulnerable population. The IRB will review and discuss essential documents relating to the trial and determine the impact the trial will have on the study population within their regulatory area. IRBs often form part of academic institutions such as Universities or Colleges; however, privately established IRBs review research affiliated with nonacademic sites/staff or organizations (IECs). Regardless of the status of the regulatory boards, all IRB's must be registered with a national body to ensure that review procedures are standardized in relation with global processes and national regulations. Furthermore, all IRBs reviewing multicenter clinical trials (especially if conducted through a US federal Department/agency) should apply for Federal Wide Assurance (FWA). FWA is an assurance of compliance with the US federal regulations for the protection of human subjects in research.

The review process is predominantly an interactive discussion between committee members, the principal investigator, and/or sponsor. Once all queries have been resolved and the IRB has sufficient evidence to support the approval of a study, the sponsor/investigator will receive written instruction that the study may commence and the period for which the study is approved.

The procedures for the IRB review may vary slightly by way of IRB composition and review procedures; however, ICH-GCP and Declaration of Helsinki (2013) remain fundamental to any IRB's Standard Operating Procedures (SOPs).

Some Useful Tips

- The applicant should confirm with the PI of the site or the institution, which HREC is representative of their area or state.
- Ensure that the HREC has a registration number and offers FWA.
- Contact the HREC to confirm submission deadlines, meeting dates, and submission fees to adequately plan trial budgets and timelines.
- Request the SOPs of the HREC to confirm submission requirements and format of the submission.
- Pay careful attention to documents requiring signature from institutional representatives prior to submission to the HREC as this too may impact on deadlines.

SOUTH AFRICA (MCC, HREC, PROVINCIAL/HOSPITAL)

The Medicines Control Council (MCC) is the national, statutory body responsible for the regulation of clinical trials and registration of medicines in South Africa. The CTA (known as the CTF1) is submitted to and reviewed by an MCC expert Clinical Trials Committee (CTC), which evaluates the scientific, medical, and ethical aspects of the application.

The HRECs in South Africa are registered with and governed by the National Health Research Ethics Committee (NHREC), this national statutory body is responsible for giving direction on ethical issues relating to health and to develop guidelines for the conduct of research involving humans subjects in South Africa. The NHREC also maintains that all ongoing research in South Africa (with the exception of Phase 1 clinical trials) must be registered on the South African National Clinical Trial Registry (SANCTR), which is accessible to the general public. The HREC reviews clinical trials in accordance with the global guidelines as well as specific South African GCP, which emphasizes review of a study with regard to vulnerable participants, placebo care, and posttrial access among other ethical considerations.

In addition to applying for approval from the MCC and HREC, all clinical trials must obtain site-specific provincial and/or hospital approval. The purpose of which is to assess the impact the clinical trial will have on the resources of the establishment in which the trial is to be conducted (staff, space, equipment, supplies, etc.). The submission requirements differ for each provincial health committee and can be found on the National Health Research Committee Website. Generally, the sponsor/investigator is required to complete a document, which stipulates the resources to be used at the trial site. This together with additional documents is submitted via an online portal or as in the case of hospital directly to the site director or superintendent for review and final approval.

Some Useful Tips
- When conducting a clinical trial in South Africa, ensure that the PI is a South African-based scientist in accordance with SAGCP (2006).
- For the MCC to approve a PI on a study, they must have sufficient experience in clinical trials as reflected on their submission CV within 2 years of the submission date.
- Applicant completing MCC submissions should pay special attention to posttrial access to investigational drug, participant reimbursement, and emergency procedures.
- Ensure that the trial obtains a DoH number from http://www.ethicsapp.co.za/ and http://www.sanctr.gov.za/ as is required for submission to MCC and HREC.
- If the study is being conducted within the provincial day hospital/clinic, the study must be registered at http://nhrd.hst.org.za/ upon receipt of ethics approval. However, if the study is being conducted in a tertiary hospital, contact the Hospital Superintendent to confirm submission requirements.

THE UNITED STATES (FDA, IRB)

CTAs for registration of medicines are submitted to the Food and Drug Administration (FDA), which operates within the US Department of Health & Human Services (DHHS) and is responsible for protecting the public health by assuring the safety, efficacy, and security of human and veterinary drugs, biological products, medical devices, food supply, and cosmetics. The FDA staff will review the submissions for clinical trials in accordance with the Federal Food, Drug, and Cosmetic Act and Code of Federal Regulations (CFR) (specifically section 21). CTAs are submitted to the FDA's Centre for Drug Evaluation and Research (CDER) through an IND application, which is submitted at the beginning of a products clinical development program and continuously updated throughout phase development. The IND application is submitted by completing the FDA 1571 and 1572 forms and all protocols associated with this product will be submitted under this IND submission. The sponsor can proceed with a clinical trial 30 days after submission of an IND application should the FDA not raise any comments.

The Office for Human Research Protections (OHRP) is a division of the Department of Health and Human Services (DHHS) with which all IRBs must be registered when reviewing research involving human subjects. In addition, OHRP works to ensure that human subjects outside of the United States who participate in research projects conducted or federally funded by DHHS or National Institute of Health (NIH) receive an equal level of protection as the research subjects inside the United States. IRBs registered with OHRP will review clinical research in accordance with FDA Regulations, ICH-GCP, and the Declaration of Helsinki, and these review procedures will be documented within the IRB-specific SOPs.

In accordance with the FDA Administration Amendments Act 801, all "applicable clinical drug trials" (this does not apply to Phase 1 trials) must be registered and updated by either the sponsor or the principal investigator on the global registry, known as www.clinicaltrials.gov. The Register is a service of the US NIH put in place to make information regarding clinical trials available to the general public. By registering the trial, the applicant will receive a National Clinical Trial (NCT) number, which should accompany the submission of an FDA3674 form to the FDA to ensure compliance with the national registry.

Some Useful Tips

- the FDA also offers an opportunity of an Pre-IND meeting allowing the applicant to engage with members of the FDA prior to submission
- The applicant can submit multiple protocols for the same product under the IND application, which should be updated annually.
- Non-US sites conducting a trial submitted as a IND are also subject to FDA regulations and therefore it is advisable to split the study into two arms and separate the protocol into two "sister studies which are operationally separate but analyzed together."

EUROPE (EMA, IRB)

Clinical trials in Europe are regulated by the European Medicines Agency (EMA) in relation with the European Commission and its Member States. Application requirements to conduct clinical trials in the EU were originally provided for in the European Directive 2001/20/EC, 2001/83/EC, and the Commission Directive 2005/28/EC, respectively. More recently, the Clinical Trials Regulation (CTR) EU No. 536/2014 has been implemented, which encompasses the legal form of afore-mentioned directives. The new CTR will ensure that the rules for conducting clinical trials are identical throughout the EU by aiming to streamline the application procedures, assessment, reporting procedures, and transparency as well as updating and enforcing GCP and GMP guidelines.

The CTA process will require that the applicant to obtain a unique EudraCT number from the EudraCT Community Clinical Trial System by registering the trial on the EU database. Once the EU number is obtained, the Investigational Medicinal Product Dossier (IMPD) or CTA will be submitted in accordance with CTR EU No. 536/2014 via the Common European Submission Portal (CESP), which will be relayed to the respective Member State for review. In this way the portal will act as a single entry point to facilitate the application and assessment of clinical data between the sponsor, the member state, regulatory bodies, and the general public. The applicant will have to register an organization and/or a user to gain access to the CESP portal and upload all documents electronically.

The applicable CTA documents will be relayed to a registered IRB who will review the protocol in accordance with the national law of the Member state concerned within the overall timelines defined by the CTR. It is only once authorization is received from the national MRA concerned and there has been a vote in favor from a registered Ethics Committee of the same member state that written confirmation of approval will be sent to the applicant allowing for study start-up.

Some Useful Tips
- Before submitting through the CESP portal, the applicant must first familiarize themselves with the Clinical Trial Regulation (CTR) EU No. 536/2014, as well as the respective member state regulations to ensure compliance of regulatory submission.

THE UNITED KINGDOM (MHRA, HRA)

The Medicine and Healthcare Products Regulatory Agency (MHRA) and more specifically the Clinical Trials Unit assesses applications to conduct clinical trials in the United Kingdom. The clinical trial authorization process requires applicants to download the application form from the Integrated Research Application System (IRAS), which enables multiple application forms to be created for review bodies providing approvals/permissions for health and social/community care research in the United Kingdom. The IRAS system will prepopulate documents throughout the submission process, and these documents in turn will be forwarded to the appropriate review boards. The IRAS system works similarly to the one point entry system of the EU portal, however, to a smaller scale. Alternatively, a clinical trial submissions can also be made through CESP, which submits the required information to the appropriate MHRA as stated in the previous section.

In addition to submitting to the MHRA, the study will also require Health Research Authorization (HRA) (this can also be done via the IRAS system), the HRA comprises a review of the clinical trial by a NHS registered Research Ethics Committee (REC). Apart from limited specific situations, only one REC needs to review a project for the whole of the United Kingdom.

AUSTRALIA (TGA, HREC, INSTITUTION/ORGANIZATIONAL APPROVAL)

There are two schemes under which clinical trials involving unapproved therapeutic goods may be conducted in Australia: (1) Clinical Trial Notification (CTN) Scheme and (2) the Clinical Trial Exemption (CTX) Scheme. The choice of which route to use (CTN or CTX) is determined by the sponsor and then by the respective Human Research Ethics Committee (HREC). These two schemes provide approval for the import, export, or supply of goods used solely for experimental purposes in Australia and which are not included in the Australian Registry of Therapeutic Goods (ARTG).

The applicant must be registered on the TGA Business Services and obtains a client ID. Once registered, the sponsor/investigator can login and complete the CTN form. The CTN form will be submitted to and signed off and approved by the HREC and the institutional "Approving Authority" after which the Sponsor will upload the CTN form and all material relating to the proposed trial to TGA Business Service.

The CTX scheme is followed for specifically high-risk studies of which very limited safety information is available (i.e., Phase I and Phase II a studies). Under the CTX scheme, the sponsor will submit a CTA directly to the TGA for review. The TGA delegate may then raise queries, which will be submitted to HREC and only once resolved will a notification be sent to TGA. Under the CTX scheme, any number of clinical trials can occur with regard to the imported TGA approved IMP (within the approved usage guidelines); however, each protocol will still require separate approval from the HREC and Approving Authority, respectively, via a CTN application.

HRECs are registered with the Australian Health Ethics Committee (AHEC), a branch of the national statutory body overseeing review policies and processes of all registered HRECs.

Lastly, prior to the enrollment of any participants on an approved trial, it is the applicants responsibility to ensure that the trail has been registered and updated on the Australian and New Zealand Clinical Trials Registry (ANZCTR).

Some Useful Tips

- The sponsor of a clinical trial in Australia must be an Australian Entity, that is, CRO, Institution, and investigator.
- The applicant should confirm with the PI of the site or the institution which HREC is representative of their area or state as well as the respective Approving Authority.
- The HREC can also be the Approving Authority for a particular trial site. The same person can sign on behalf of the HREC and the Approving Authority but they should indicate their position or capacity in relation to each.

CHINA (CFDA, CDE, HOSPITAL/INSTITUTION, IRB)

There are various regulatory bodies in China; however, all CTAs (including bioequivalence studies) will be submitted to the China, Food and Drug Administration (CFDA) [previously known as the State Food and Drug Administration (SFDA)] for registration. The CFDA designates previously approved drugs as category III "import drugs" and requires clinical data from Phase I through Phase III clinical trials conducted in China to support an application for an import drug license. This is the only option for drugs already marketed in another country. However, for drugs that have not yet been approved anywhere elsewhere, applicants can choose to conduct a full clinical development program in China and submit a category I New Drug Application (NDA) in an attempt to earn market approval sooner. The sponsors must submit a CTA to the CFDA for review, which includes review by the Centre for Drug Evaluation (CDE), the National Institutes of Food and Drug Control (NIFDC), and the Centre of Food and Drug Inspection (CFDI).

The CDE, NIFDC, and CFDI will review and conduct an on-site inspection of the submitted CTA and perform sample testing of the new medicine to confirm the authenticity, precision, and integrity of the dossier submitted. The CDE's review will submit a Clinical Trial Permit (CTP) to the CFDA for confirmation and approval. The CFDA approval process of the CTP is a lengthy process spanning up to an additional 18 months after the initial CTA submission. Following approval from the CFDA, regulatory reporting and subsequent submission will be at a FDA Provincial Level.

In addition, a clinical trial can only be carried out in China if the study design is approved from an overseeing ethics review board (IRB/EC). IRBs in China have been split into Central Ethics Committee registered with the CFDA and Institutional Ethics Committees which form part of registered hospitals and research institutions. Although regulations are unclear of which IRB the submission must be submitted to, it is suggested that for multicenter trials submission be made to central ethics committee, which can then be forwarded to the institutional ethics committee.

Lastly, the approved clinical trial must be conducted in CFDA-certified research institutions/hospitals that operate in compliance with Chinese GCP.

Some Useful Tips
- Ethics reviews can be initiated before the CFDAs issue the CTP.
- It is advised that an applicant submitting a study for the first time in China team up with international CROs (multicenter trials) or domestic CROs (collaborative research) to ensure that submissions are done in accordance with regulatory requirements and prevent any delays.
- It is suggested that CTA application be submitted to the central ethics committee for the scientific review and the institutional ethics committees to coordinate continuing review processes.

INDIA (DCGI, CDSCO, IEC)

India's equivalent Medical Research Authority is the office of the Drugs Controller General India (DCGI). Clinical trials are regulated per Schedule Y of the Drug and Cosmetics Act (1940) and Drug Cosmetic Rules (DCR), 2005 and 1945. Due to significant delays in approval timelines, clinical trials have been divided into two categories, namely Category A and Category B. Category A trials are clinical trials, which have received approval from regulatory agencies in nine regions of the World (i.e., the United States, the United Kingdom, Switzerland, Australia, Canada, Germany, South Africa, Japan, and Europe). These submissions have an increased turn-around time for approval while Category B trials often take much longer as they have not received approval from these recognized international MRAs.

The Central Drug Standard Control Organization (CDSCO) is a Department of the Ministry of Health that handles the approval process of clinical trials specifically and to whom the CTA's are submitted. CDSCO has launched a system to allow online submission and monitoring of CTAs, which requires the input of information for the sponsor/CRO, Investigator, Ethics Committee, and clinical trial subjects. The sponsor/investigator is to complete Form 44 and submit the CTA dossier to CDSCO for review.

In addition to obtaining approval from CDSCO, it is now and established mandatory requirement that it is the sponsor/investigator's responsibility to register and update the trial on the national Clinical Trials Registry- India (CTRI) for public access.

All sites must obtain IEC approval from and IEC registered by an appropriate licensing authority established under the DCGIs. Similar to global requirements, the IEC must prepare a constitution and SOPs for its operation, which can be requested by the investigator/sponsor in preparation of a submission.

Some Useful Tips

- CTA submissions to CDSCO can now be submitted via an online submission platform at http://octams.gov.in.
- Submission of IEC and DCGI approval is essential for trial registration in the CTRI.
- Submissions to CDSCO and IEC can be done in parallel.

CONCLUSION

Regulatory bodies are responsible for ensuring the protection and safety of the population and to ensure the high quality of trial data. It is clear that the regulation of clinical trials is an extensive and time consuming endeavor shared by both national and provincial representatives. Although each country has its own regulatory systems in place for conducting an IND trial, similarities in review process and the prerequisites are evident. These similarities include (1) the approval from the national MRA or delegated representative committee, (2) the approval from a registered IRB/IEC, (3) the approval from the institution/site where the trial will take place, and finally, (4) the registration of the trial on the national registry/database accessible to the general public. Interestingly, the requirement of having to register a clinical trial on registries accessible to the public is being enforced by various publication entities. For publication purposes, authors of clinical trial protocols are now required to submit the registration number provided by the national database for the publishing of the trial results. The clinical industry is competitive and lucrative field with the first sponsor product producing positive results having the opportunity to submit a NDA for the registration and marketing of the drug to the same regulatory body. It is therefore in the best interest of the applicant, whether it be the investigator or the sponsor, that they are intimately familiar with the regulatory requirements and understand the legislation enforcing these requirements to prevent any delays in the approval process by these regulatory bodies.

FURTHER READING

Guidance for Industry; E6 good clinical practice: consolidated guidance, ICH April 2006.

World Medical Association. Declaration of Helsinki Ethical Principles for Medical Research Involving Human Subjects. JAMA 2013;310(20):2191−4. Available from: http://dx.doi.org/10.1001/jama.2013.281053.

South Africa

Department of Health. Guidelines for good clinical practice in conduct of clinical trials with human participants in South Africa. Pretoria, South Africa: Department of Health; 2006.

Medicine Control Council; publications; application forms; document 6.05 CTF1 May03 v1.doc; May 2003. Avaliable from http://www.mccza.com/Publications/Index/8 [accessed 22.11.16].

Medicine Control Council; publications; clinical trials document 2.12_Completing_CT_applications_May03_v1_1.doc; May 2003. Available from http://www.mccza.com/Publications/Index/6 [accessed 22.11.16].

National Health Research Electronic Application System (NHREC); home page. Available from www.ethicsapp.co.za [accessed 22.11.16].

Department of Health, Republic of South Africa. South African Clinical Trial Register (SANCTR). Available from http://www.sanctr.gov.za/InvestigatorInformation/Howtoregister/tabid/180/Default.aspx [accessed 22.11.16].

Department of Health, Republic of South Africa. National Health research Ethics Council. Available from http://www.nhrec.org.za/ [accessed 22.11.16].

National Health Research Database (NHRD): Provincial Health Research Committees (PHRCs). Available from http://nhrd.hst.org.za/Home/Resources [accessed 22.11.16].

The United States

U.S Food and Drug Administration; drugs development & approval process (drugs), how drugs are developed and approved types of applications: investigational new drug (IND) application. Available from http://www.fda.gov/Drugs/DevelopmentApprovalProcess/HowDrugsareDevelopedandApproved/ApprovalApplications/InvestigationalNewDrugINDApplication/default.htm [accessed 22.11.16].

Department of Health and Human Services; Office of Human Research Protection. Available from http://www.hhs.gov/ohrp/about-ohrp/index.html# [accessed 22.11.16].

ClinicalTrials.gov. Available from https://clinicaltrials.gov/ct2/manage-recs/fdaaa [accessed 22.11.16].

EMA

European Medicines Association; Clinical trials. Available from http://www.ema.europa.eu/ema/index.jsp?curl = pages/special_topics/general/general_content_000489.jsp&mid = WC0b01ac058060676f [accessed 22.11.16].

EUDraCT. Available from https://eudract.ema.europa.eu/ [accessed 22.11.16].

European Medicine Association; Clinical trial regulations. Available from http://www.ema.europa.eu/ema/index.jsp?curl = pages/regulation/general/general_content_000629.jsp&mid = WC0b01ac05808768df/ [accessed 22.11.16].

HMA: Common European submission Portal. Available from https://cespportal.hma.eu/Account/Login [accessed 22.1116].

http://ec.europa.eu/health/human-use/clinical-trials/information/index_en.htm#ct2.

The United Kingdom

Gov.UK: Clinical trials for medicines: apply for authorisation in the UK. Available from https://www.gov.uk/guidance/clinical-trials-for-medicines-apply-for-authorisation-in-the-uk [accessed 22.11.16].

Australia

Australian Government: Department of Health: Therapeutic goods administration: industry: regulation basics: clinical trials. Available from https://www.tga.gov.au/form/ctn-scheme-forms [accessed 22.11.16].

Australian Government: Department of Health: Therapeutic goods administration: home: industry: regulation basics: clinical trials: CTN scheme forms. Available from https://www.tga.gov.au/getting-started-online-ctn-form [accessed 22.11.16].

Australian Government: Department of Health: Therapeutic goods administration: home: industry: regulation basics: clinical trials: CTX scheme forms. Available from https://www.tga.gov.au/form/ctx-scheme-forms [accessed 22.11.16].

Australian Government: Department of Health: Therapeutic goods administration: home: industry: regulation basics: clinical trials: Human Research Ethics Committees and the therapeutic goods legislation. Available from https://www.tga.gov.au/publication/human-research-ethics-committees-and-therapeutic-goods-legislation [accessed 22.11.16].

Australian Government: National Health and Medical Research Council (NHMRC): home: health and research ethics Human Research Ethics Committees (HRECs). Available from https://www.nhmrc.gov.au/health-ethics/human-research-ethics-committees-hrecs [accessed 22.11.16].

China

China FDA: Home: laws and regulations: Available from http://eng.sfda.gov.cn/WS03/CL0768/61645.html [accessed 22.11.16].

China FDA. Available from http://www.sfda.gov.cn/WS01/CL0412/ [accessed 22.11.16].

India

Central Drugs Standard Control Organization: Home: for industry: checklist for pre-screening of application: 3. Clinical trial and new drug applications. Available from http://www.cdsco.nic.in/forms/list.aspx?lid=2053&Id=3 [accessed 22.11.16].

Central Drugs Standard Control Organization: Home: for industry: checklist for pre-screening of application: 15. Global clinical trial checklist. Available from http://www.cdsco.nic.in/forms/list.aspx?lid=2053&Id=3 [accessed 22.11.16].

Central Drugs Standard Control Organization: Home: new drugs: 13. Draft guidance on approval of clinical trials & new drug. Available from http://www.cdsco.nic.in/writereaddata/Guidance_for_New_Drug_Approval-23.07.2011.pdf [accessed 22.11.16].

Clinical Trials: Online trial application and monitoring system. Available from https://octams.gov.in/about [accessed 22.11.16].

Clinical Trials Registry India: National Institute of Medical statistics: Indian Council of Medical Research. Available from http://ctri.nic.in/Clinicaltrials/login.php [accessed 22.11.16].

Morulaa Health Tech. Available from http://www.morulaa.com/indian-medical-device-market/clinical-trials-in-india-document-requirements/ [accessed 22.11.16].

Chapter 5

Contracts and Agreements

Brenda Wright

Chapter Outline

There are usually many parties involved in the conduct of a clinical trial and the contracts and agreements should make clear reference to what is expected of each party. These contracts/agreements may be internal or external and both legal or nonlegal.

All contracts and agreements in a clinical trial should be agreed to and signed by all parties prior to the start of any trial. These contracts must be reviewed and updated to ensure that they remain relevant and up to date. All changes must be documented timeously and signed by all parties involved.

> ICH-GCP E6 Section 1: *A contract is a written, dated signed agreement between two parties that sets out any arrangements on delegation and distribution of tasks and obligations and, if appropriate, on financial matters. The protocol may serve as basis of a contract.*

The content of agreements and contracts will have the following guidelines:

1. Procedures to be performed in the conduct of the trial.
2. The lines of communication that should be followed during the trial.

A Comprehensive and Practical Guide to Clinical Trials.
DOI: http://dx.doi.org/10.1016/B978-0-12-804729-3.00005-5

3. The roles and responsibilities of all parties involved during the clinical trial.
4. The Clinical Trial Regulations standards as applicable.

CLINICAL TRIAL AGREEMENT/SITE AGREEMENT

This agreement is signed between the Sponsor and the legal entity of the site that will conduct the trial. This could be the legal department of academic institutions. (Principal Investigator signs as third party or acknowledgment of agreement.)

There are standard contract terms that should always be described in the Clinical Trial Agreement (CTA):

Parties to the Agreement

The roles and responsibilities of the Principal Investigator should be documented in the CTA. If the trial is conducted at multisites, each Principal Investigator should understand their particular responsibilities and the allocation of all trial tasks should be documented in the CTA.

Study Details

The protocol should always be incorporated by reference into the contract.

> ICH-GCP Section 5.6.2: *Before entering in an agreement with an investigator/institution to conduct a clinical trial, the sponsor should provide the investigator/institution with the protocol and an updated Investigator's Brochure, and should provide sufficient time for the investigator/institution to review the protocol and the information provided.*

Compliance

Compliance to: protocol, International Council for Harmonization-Good Clinical Practice (ICH-GCP) guidelines, ethical approval obtained, professional standards, identified standard operating procedures, accurate data recording, safe storage of records and provision for monitoring, audits and ongoing cooperation, and liaison between parties.

Timelines

Start date and duration/end date should be described in the CTA. Number of subjects to be recruited by specific dates and options if recruitment dates are not on target should be mentioned as well. Timelines regarding status reports, providing interim analysis reports and submitting the final report should be described.

Data Confidentiality and Safe and Secure Storage of Data

Data should be kept confidential and safety and security of data must be maintained. Archiving should be consistent with ICH-GCP guidelines, the rights to access, removal, or delivery of data and materials should be specified.

Data Intellectual Property Must be Described

The following details regarding intellectual property should be specified in the CTA:

1. Protection and Intellectual Property rights of the Sponsor.
2. Investigator's intellectual property.
3. The investigator's right to publish.

Indemnity and Compensation

Indemnity should be provided by the Sponsor before the start of the study against any loss incurred by the investigator as a result of claims arising from the trial.

Indemnity should also be provided by the contracted research organization (CRO) or Investigator in favor of the sponsor in respect of negligence, malpractice, or breach of contract by the CRO or investigator.

Financial provision for handling claims should be described in the agreement (e.g., insurance arrangements).

Insurance

Sponsor must ensure that insurance is in place to cover its liability and that of the Investigator or the sponsor should provide evidence of financial resources regarding liability.

Investigator/Institution must ensure that he/she/it has liability insurance (in case of neglect).

Termination

Appropriate provision for termination must be made on specific grounds, rights of termination, and termination upon insolvency, administration, or liquidation of either party.

General

1. The law of the country that is to govern the agreement should be stipulated.

2. Submission to the jurisdiction of the courts of a particular country in relation to disputes.
3. Notice-methods of affecting notice and contact points.
4. Signature of contract by authorized signatories.

Payment

ICH-GCP Section 5.9: *Financial aspects of a trial should be documented in an agreement between the sponsor and the investigator/institution.*

The agreed budget between the site/Principal Investigator and the Sponsor/funder should form part of this agreement and should specify the following:

1. The amounts and timing of payments.
2. Separate accounts to be established.
3. Provision for alteration of budget if there is an amendment to the protocol, and extend of services to be provided as well as early termination.

SOME EXAMPLES OF OTHER CONTRACTS

Cosponsorship Agreement

A cosponsorship agreement defines the legal responsibilities of the parties involved in the clinical trial. This agreement is signed between the cosponsors of a clinical trial, for example, an agreement between a national funding agent and a university.

Funding Agreement

A Funding Agreement relates to the terms and conditions related to the funds granted and is signed between the funder of the clinical trial (usually investigator lead trials) and the Principal Investigator.

Collaboration Agreements

Pharmaceutical companies sign collaboration agreements for new products in their pipelines and biotech companies to access the resources needed for final stage development, clinical trials, manufacturing, and distribution.

Intellectual Property Agreements

These contracts are signed between collaborating institutions and describes the rights associated with the intellectual property and the purchase and sale of intellectual property rights that may be created during the term of the collaboration.

Service Level Agreements

These Agreements are signed with external suppliers such as central laboratories, external statisticians, and central database centers.

Material Transfer Agreements

A material transfer agreement (MTA) is a contract that governs the transfer of tangible research materials between two organizations, when the recipient intends to use it for his/her own research purposes. The MTA defines the rights of the provider and the recipient with respect to the materials and any derivatives. This agreement will describe the handling requirements for material (e.g., tissue samples that is transferred from trial site to various laboratories).

Pharmacy Technical Agreements

This agreement covers processes applied to investigative medicinal product such as packaging, manufacture, and labeling.

Keypoints

- *ICH-GCP E6 Section 1*: "A contract is a written, dated signed agreement between two parties that sets out any arrangements on delegation and distribution of tasks and obligations and, if appropriate, on financial matters. The protocol may serve as basis of a contract."

  There are standard contract terms that should always be described in the CTA:
- parties to agreement,
- study details,
- compliance,
- responsibilities,
- timelines,
- data, confidentiality,
- insurance/indemnity,
- termination,
- general,
- payment.

FURTHER READING

Guidance for Industry, E6 (R1) Good clinical practice: consolidated guidance, April 1996, accessed February 2016.

http://www.ct-toolkit.ac.uk/routemap/archiving [accessed October 2016].

Chapter 6

Protocol, Informed Consent Documents, and Investigator Brochure

Brenda Wright

Chapter Outline

PROTOCOL

- Conducting a clinical trial is similar to baking a soufflé. If you do not follow the recipe in detail, your soufflé will not be a success. Or, if the recipe lacks detail or ingredients, the end product will also be unsuccessful. In clinical research the protocol is our "recipe." It should have all the ingredients necessary to know what, when, and how to conduct the trial. The key to success in conducting a clinical trial is a well-written detailed protocol.

- A protocol describes the conduct of a clinical trial (i.e., the methodology, design, objectives, and the statistical considerations). It also describes the safety management and reporting of the trial subjects and the integrity of the data collected.

- In this section of this chapter, we look at what is required in a clinical trial protocol as described in the ICH E6 Section 6 guidelines. These guidelines also mention site-specific information that may be addressed in a separate agreement, and that some of the information required may be contained in other protocol referenced documents, such as an Investigator's Brochure.

- The CONSORT (CONsolidated Standards of Reporting Trials) 2010 guideline is a good reference to visit when designing your protocol for a parallel-group randomized controlled trial [1]. This guideline discusses

A Comprehensive and Practical Guide to Clinical Trials.
DOI: http://dx.doi.org/10.1016/B978-0-12-804729-3.00006-7

trial design, the conduct of the trial, the analysis and interpretation of the trial, and the validity of its results.

1. *General Information* in a protocol should contain the following:
   a. Protocol Title, Protocol Number, Protocol Date, and Protocol Version.
   b. Name and address of the sponsor/CRO.
   c. Name and title of Principal Investigator, address and contact details of site unless the trial is conducted at multisites.
   d. Name and address(es) of laboratories/technical departments or other institutions involved.
   e. Protocol synopsis—The synopsis is a summary of your protocol and should provide a broad overview of your protocol details such as: title, investigational sites, study number, final protocol, objectives, study design, inclusion/exclusion criteria, dose and mode of administration of investigative medicinal product (IMP), study duration, endpoints, sample size, and statistical analysis.

2. *Background Information and Scientific Rationale* include the following:
   a. Name and descriptions of the investigational product as well as the justification for the route of administration, dosage, dosage regimen, and treatment periods.
   b. Statement of compliance with the protocol, GCP, and the applicable regulatory requirements.
   c. Description of the population to be studied.
   d. Summaries of potential risks and benefits and why the value of the information to be gained outweighs the risks involved. Note: Payment to participants is not considered as a "benefit" but rather a reimbursement for money spent on traveling and time.
   e. Relevant references to literature and data that provide background for the trial.

3. *Trial Objectives and Purpose* are the reason for performing a study in terms of the scientific question to be answered by analysis of the data collected and should have the following details described:
   a. Primary and secondary objectives of the study.
   b. Primary outcome measures (end points). Normally there will only be one primary observation/variable, with evidence that it will provide a clinically relevant, valid and reliable measure of the primary objective.
   c. Secondary outcome measures (end points). These are supportive information related to the disease/research question.

4. *Trial Design*
   ICH-GCP Section 6.4: "The scientific integrity of the trial and the credibility of the data from the trial depend substantially on the trial design." The design should include:

a. Specific Primary and Secondary endpoints to be measured during the trial.
b. Type/design of trial to be conducted (e.g., double-blind, placebo controlled, open-label, dose escalation) as well as the phase of the trial and if single or multisites will be participating. A schematic diagram of trial design, procedures, and stages should be included. See example from CONSORT guideline in Fig. 6.1 [1].

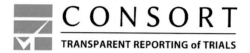

CONSORT 2010 Flow Diagram

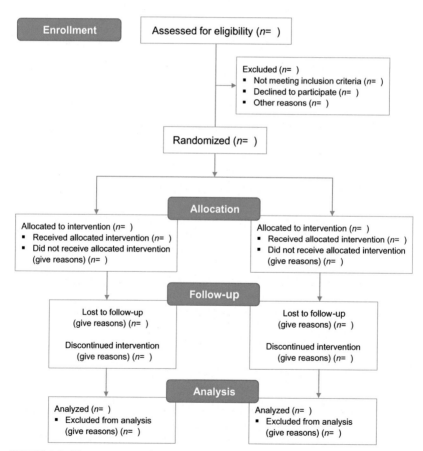

FIGURE 6.1   Transparent reporting of trials.

c. The study populations (e.g., healthy participants, sick patients, inpatient/outpatient), sample size, and expected duration of subject participation.

d. Detailed randomization and blinding description where applicable. (To minimize/avoid bias.)

e. "Stopping rules" or "discontinuation criteria" for individual participants.

f. The study plan:

The study plan should be illustrated by a study flowchart (see Chapter 7, Planning, Fig. 7.2) as well as a detailed description of all study procedures and visits, evaluations to be done, procedures for administrating the study product or intervention, follow-up procedures, and visits after administration. Define when the final study visit should occur as well as procedures/evaluations to be performed and instructions to be given to the participant. Remember to include the early termination visits and unscheduled visits and describe details and evaluations required during these visits.

g. Eligibility criteria:

Should provide a definition of subject characteristics required to be enrolled in the study. Inclusion/Exclusion criteria should be designed based on the risks of the test agent/product. Screening laboratory tests should be selected to evaluate safety, with ranges based on toxicity criteria.

h. The treatment of participants should be described in detail:

   i. Names of products, acquisition, formulation, packaging, labeling, and product storage and stability—these could also be referenced to the pharmacy manual.

   ii. Dosage, preparation, and administration of IMP/device.

   iii. Accountability procedures.

   iv. Procedures for monitoring participant compliance.

   v. Prohibited medications/treatments before and during the trial. (Ensure that these are consistent with the ones listed in the inclusion/exclusion criteria.)

   vi. Withdrawal times of concomitant medication and/or treatments where applicable.

   vii. Rescue treatments or medications that are included in the study design.

5. *Assessment of Safety*

   a. List all safety parameters that are outcome measures.

   b. Include other parameters if not primary/secondary study outcome measures.

   c. Adverse Events, Serious Adverse Events, Expected and Unexpected Adverse Reactions should be described in detail. This includes: definitions, severity, relation to study product, actions taken, outcomes and reporting structures, and individual responsible for each step (e.g., the investigator, the medical monitor). It should also include which forms should be completed, how reports will be distributed and what follow-up is required.

    d. Include halting rules.

6. *Statistics*

    a. Study hypotheses; describe the hypotheses for primary and key secondary objectives, specifying the type of comparison (e.g., equivalence, dose-response, superiority, or noninferiority).

    b. Provide all information needed to validate your calculations.

    c. Planned Interim Analysis (if applicable); describe the composition and how often meetings will take place if the interim analysis will be reviewed by a Data Safety Monitoring Board (DSMB) or similar committee.

    d. The final analysis plan should discuss how outcome measures will be assessed and transformed, if relevant, before analysis.

7. *Administrative*

    a. Specify in protocol that the Investigator/Institution will permit trial-related monitoring, audits, Institutional Review Board (IRB)/Independent Ethics Committees (IEC) review, and regulatory inspections.

    b. Site will maintain appropriate medical and research records in compliance with ICH-GCP E6, Section 4.9 and regulatory and institutional requirements for the protection of confidentiality of participants.

    c. Quality Control and Quality Assurance will be performed throughout the conduct of the trial.

8. *Ethics, Regulatory, and Legal*

    a. Include the guiding ethical principles to be followed during the conduct of the trial.

    b. Protocol, amendments, associated informed consent documents, and recruitment material will be reviewed and approved by an appropriate IRB/IEC prior to use.

    c. Describe procedures for maintaining participant confidentiality, any special data security requirements, and retention of records.

9. *Data Handling and Record Keeping*

    a. Describe methods to ensure that data collected are accurate, consistent, complete, and reliable, and in accordance with ICH E6. This includes reference to source documents, case report forms, instructions for completing forms, data handling procedures, and data-monitoring procedures.

    b. Provide details regarding data capturing—specify if paper or electronic.

    c. Indicate timelines for data review and reports.

    d. Specify the length of time documents are to be kept and destruction details after time period has elapsed.

  e. Describe the reporting and documentation of protocol violations and noncompliance.

10. *Publication Policy*

  Reference to the Clinical Trial Agreement or Specific Grant must be made regarding the publication and authorship policies.

11. *Literature References*

  Include a list of relevant references in your protocol.

INFORMED CONSENT

Informed consent for a clinical trial consists of two parts: a signed document and the process of obtaining consent. It is an ongoing process that must occur prior to any trial-related procedures are conducted as well as during the conduct of the trial.

  The Clinical Trial Informed Consent Document is a summary of the trial. This document should be written in "laymen" terms, that is, easy to understand by the nonresearch public and age related. It should include the purpose of the trial, the treatment procedures, and schedule of events. Potential risks and benefits and participant rights should be discussed as well as alternative treatments.

1. *Informed Consent Guidelines*

  a. ICH-GCP Section 1.28 describes the informed consent process. The requirements and process for obtaining informed consent from a clinical trial participant can be found in Section 4.8.

  b. There are also national and local regulatory requirements, sponsor requirements, and personal data security regulations applicable in the country in which the study is being conducted to take into consideration.

  c. The informed consent documents must be approved by an IRB or IEC prior to its use.

  d. The Council for International Organisations for Medical Sciences (CIOMS) has one of the most advanced international guidelines regarding the informed consent process.

  e. This guideline states: "obtaining informed consent is a process that is begun when initial contact is made with a prospective subject and continues throughout the course of the study. By informing the prospective subjects, by repetition and explanation, by answering their questions as they arise, and by ensuring that each individual understands each procedure, investigators elicit their informed consent and in doing so manifest respect for their dignity and autonomy. Each individual must be given as much time as is needed to reach a decision, including time for consultation with family. Informing the individual subject must not be simply a ritual recitation of the contents of a written document. Rather, the investigator must convey the informa-tion ... in language that suits the individual's level of understanding ... the investigator must then ensure that the prospective subject has adequately understood the information."

2. *Informed Consent Process*
    a. The Principal Investigator (PI) may delegate the task of administering and obtaining informed consent to a qualified individual; however, he or she is ultimately responsible for ensuring the process is conducted properly.
    b. The PI/delegate discusses the trial's risks, benefits, and other aspects with the potential participant and, if required, the participant's legal representative, before the trial begins.
    c. The PI gives the potential participant ample time and opportunity to ask questions about the trial and discuss it with relatives and family members.
    d. If the potential participant decides to get involved in the trial, he or she provides voluntary consent by signing and dating the written-informed consent document of which he or she also receives a copy. The participant has the right to withdraw consent at any time without penalty, repercussions, or reason.
    e. The consent process should be documented in the participant's source documents. This is done by the person obtaining the consent. Details to be documented are as follows:
        - Description of how consent was obtained—written or verbally.
        - The participant's level of comprehension, that is, did the partici-pant understand the main purpose of the study, procedures to be done, risks involved in participating and frequency and duration of visits?
        - Start time and end time of consent process.
        - Questions asked by the participant and answers given.

3. *Informed Consent Document*
    a. The informed consent document must include the 20 ICH-required elements (Section 4.8.10 of the GCP guidance). As mentioned before, they will include the purpose, duration, risks, benefits, costs, and additional expenses of the trial; a description of the trial procedures; alternative care options; and volunteers' rights.
    b. The document also must have at least two signature and date lines: one for the participant and another for the health care professional conducting the informed consent discussions with the participant.
    c. Both the written document and the verbal consenting process must be presented in language the participant understands. This must be documented appropriately.
    d. Informed consent documents must be revised every time new safety information becomes available or there is a change in trial

procedures, participant compensation, or personnel noted on the consent form. Revised documents must be approved by an IRB/IEC prior to its use. The informed consent document with the new information must be discussed with the participant and signed by the relevant parties.

Never forget Principle 1 of the Nuremberg Code: "The voluntary consent of the human subject is absolutely essential."

INVESTIGATOR BROCHURE

1. The Investigational Brochure is a summary of information regarding an investigational product obtained during preclinical and other clinical trials.
2. The investigators brochure (IB) is intended to provide the investigator with details necessary to manage a clinical trial and study participants.
3. It provides the investigator information regarding possible risks and adverse reactions, and of specific precautions that may be needed.
4. The IB should also provide information regarding the recognition and treatment of overdose and the possible treatment thereof.
5. The sponsor is responsible to update the IB. It should be reviewed annually and/or whenever new and important information becomes available.
6. Key aspects addressed in the IB are:
   - dosing of the study drug,
   - methods of administration,
   - frequency of dosing intervals,
   - safety monitoring procedures.

Main sections of an IB:

1. Title page:
   Displays the Sponsor's name, the identity of the investigational product (products), an edition number and date, and the number and date of the edition it supersedes.
2. List of abbreviations.
3. Contents.
4. Summary:
   This is an overview of all subsequent sections. It is a summary of significant physical, chemical, and pharmaceutical properties of the investigational product, and also pharmacological, toxicological, pharmacokinetic, metabolic, and therapeutic information that is relevant to the appropriate stage of clinical trial.
5. Introduction:
   The introduction provides the chemical name (and generic and trade names, if approved) of the investigational product, all active components, pharmacological class, the rationale for performing further research with

the investigational product, and anticipated indications for its use. This section should provide the investigative approach to be followed in evaluating the investigational product.

6. Physical, chemical, and pharmaceutical properties and formulation:

This section provides the investigator with sufficient information so that potential risks associated with the IMP can be assessed. It also provides information regarding the handling, storage, and preparation of IMP needed, prior to administration.

7. Nonclinical studies:

ICH E6 provides a basic structure regarding this section. It lists the type of information to be summarized. The nonclinical studies section should provide the data from animal studies regarding nonclinical pharmacological, pharmacokinetic, metabolic, and toxicological characteristics of the investigational drug.

8. Effects in humans:

This section is a summary of results obtained in all previous studies conducted with the IMP. ECH E6 specifies that a summary must be completed on the pharmacokinetics, metabolism, pharmacodynamics, dose-response, safety, efficacy, and other pharmacological activities.

9. Summary of data and guidance for the investigators:

This section of the IB contains information such as therapeutic indications, contraindications, warnings, and precautions for use.

Keypoints

Study Protocol:
- The key to success in conducting a clinical trial is a well-written detailed protocol.
- Protocol should contain: general information, scientific rationale and background information, trial objectives and purpose, trial design, assessment of safety, statistics, administration, Ethics, Regulatory, and Legal requirements, Data handling and record keeping, publication policy, and references.

Informed Consent:
- Informed consent for a clinical trial consists of two parts: a signed document and the process of obtaining consent.
- It is an ongoing process that must occur prior to any trial-related procedures are conducted as well as during the conduct of the trial.
- Informed consent document should be written in "laymen" terms, that is, easy to understand by the nonresearch public and age related.
- Informed consent document should include the purpose of the trial, the treatment procedures, and schedule of events. Potential risks and benefits and participant rights should be discussed as well as alternative treatments.

(Continued)

Keypoints (Continued)

- The PI may delegate the task of administering and obtaining informed consent to a qualified individual; however, he or she is ultimately responsible for ensuring the process is conducted properly.
- The consent process should be documented in the participant's source documents.

Investigator Brochure:

- The Investigational Brochure is a summary of information regarding an investigational product obtained during preclinical and other clinical trials.
- The IB is intended to provide the investigator with details necessary to manage a clinical trial and study participants.
- Key aspects addressed in the IB are dosing of the study drug, methods of administration, frequency of dosing intervals, and safety monitoring procedures.

REFERENCE

[1]   Schulz KF, Altman DG, Moher Dfor the CONSORT Group. CONSORT 2010 Statement: updated guidelines for reporting parallel group randomised trials. Ann Int Med 2010;152 Epub 24 March.

FURTHER READING

http://www.ct-toolkit.ac.uk/routemap/archiving [accessed October 2016].
http://www.clinicaltrials.com/study_participants/informed_consent.htm.
https://www.acrpnet.org/wp/content/uploads/2016/09/ACRPWhitePaperTheProcessofInformed Consent.pdf.
http://www.medtran.ru/eng/trials/protomechanics/ch3.htm.

Chapter 7

Planning

Brenda Wright

Chapter Outline

In Chapter 6, Protocol, Informed Consent Documents, and Investigator Brochure, we discussed the documents that will supply us with information needed to conduct a clinical trial. We also looked at how to prioritize the content of these documents and who will be responsible for each section.

We can now proceed in planning the conduct of the trial. This will be supported by a fictitious case study for a typical Early Phase Trial (see Appendix 7.1: Case Study, at the end of this chapter). At this stage all regulatory documents have been submitted, contracts are in the process of being signed and we have an indication of recruitment and enrollment deadlines.

This stage of the clinical trial is not set in stone and the only certainty is that things will change as you progress. That is why it is so important to

A Comprehensive and Practical Guide to Clinical Trials.
DOI: http://dx.doi.org/10.1016/B978-0-12-804729-3.00007-9

keep track of your planning with regular updates. Communication between the team members is vital and team meetings are essential.

The following is a step-by-step process with useful templates to complete for all activities prior to, during and after completion of the conduct of a trial.

SCHEDULE OF EVENTS

The schedule of events (Appendix 7.2) in the trial protocol is a very handy tool for the trial manager. This lists exactly which events and tasks must take place. Always make sure that you check the schedule with the body of the protocol and advise the sponsor should any discrepancies occur.

DESIGN A PRETRIAL CHECKLIST

It is important to keep track of proceedings at any stage of a clinical trial. Communicating with the rest of your team members, contractors, etc., are critical. The following Prestudy checklist is an example of how to keep track of matters outstanding (Appendix 7.3). You identify team members and their responsibilities, and you can monitor progress in getting ready to start the conduct of the trial. This is a working document and you can complete and add to it as time passes.

DRAW UP A TRIAL CALENDAR

A trial calendar will assist you when planning your trial visit dates (Appendix 7.4). This way you can ensure that the visit days of different cohorts do not overlap and that it fits in with the rest of your site's activities, especially when you have to move admission dates after the trial has started. This working document will change as time progresses, as you will never know before the time exactly when you will admit all your cohorts. The only certainty about clinical trial timelines is that it will change all the time as you go along.

The example below shows the calendar for the first two cohorts from our case study. You can design this calendar in more detail if you like and add in your Start-Up Meetings (Investigator Meeting) and Site Initiation Meeting dates, your monitor visit dates, your Data Safety Monitoring Board (DSMB) meeting dates, etc. You can also add activities on your visit days, for example, Pk, safety bloods, ECG, physical exam, etc.

COMPILE A TRIAL BUDGET

Most sites will have their own finance department that will deal mostly with the contracts and cost estimates/trial budgets from sponsor companies. However, your finance department may not always know how long each trial visit will take, how many staff members you will need on certain trial days, and what consumables you may need and so it is very helpful if you prepare a cost estimate/budget from your side as well to share with them. Use the schedule of events from your protocol to calculate staff hours spent on each visit (Appendix 7.5). This is also important when you apply for a grant in the case of academic trials. You can then follow upon your expenditures/staff hours worked to make sure that you do not over-extend your budget. Talk the Clinical Team through the budget.

Appendix 7.5 is an example of a study budget. Note the interesting fact that the screen to enrollment ratio is 2:1. If you look at the status report (Appendix 7.4) for this example, you will see that 8 more were actually screened than planned (104) due to the strict inclusion/exclusion criteria. You would have to renegotiate with the sponsor to see if they would cover the costs for the additional participants screened. This ratio is something to take note of before you sign the contract with the Sponsor.

You will also notice from Appendix 7.9 that 584 participants were pre-screened. The hours that the recruitment staff had to spend contacting and speaking to these potential participants were not calculated in this budget and the budget should be updated.

Any costs that the Sponsor pays directly to external contractors, for example, Local Laboratory, Radiology Departments, specialized equipment, etc., will not be shown on this budget. The Sponsor will have separate contracts with these suppliers. Should they pay the regulatory authorities directly the fees will also not appear on this spreadsheet. Normally the remuneration to participants is a separate cost that is invoiced separately and is also not shown on this budget spreadsheet.

All this information will be stipulated in the contract. Make sure that you check the contract to identify separate costs prior to calculating your budget.

DESIGN A STAFF WORK SCHEDULE

A staff work schedule can be used to assist with determining how many staff you will need on busier days on the floor (Appendix 7.6). This schedule is color coded and shows all the activities to be conducted on a particular trial day, the time it is planned and who will be responsible. Each staff member will receive a copy of this schedule and the study coordinator will oversee the day's activities and act as a backup should staff run into trouble with late sampling, etc. As an example, the following staff schedule covers Day 1 activities of the case study.

DO STOCK LIST FOR EQUIPMENT AND CONSUMABLES

A trial-specific stock list should be drawn up and all equipment and consumables used for the trial should be listed with expiry dates where applicable

(Appendix 7.7). Expiry dates on consumables should be checked and the stock list should be updated once a month until the trial is completed. Discard any expired stock in the appropriate way (according to your local waste disposal regulations).

Copies of the calibration certificates of all equipment must be filed in the Trial Site File. Make sure that the calibration dates are valid. Most equipment needs calibration once a year, but check the manufacturers' recommendation. Sponsors must supply calibration documents with any specialized equipment they supply to the site. Do not discard any containers and/or boxes that equipment is packed in on arrival (especially specialized equipment shipped by the Sponsor) as you would have to repack and ship the equipment back to the Sponsor at the end of the trial.

All equipment and stock must be locked away in a safe place. Certain consumables like the Laboratory Kits may have to be stored at a specific temperature.

ENSURE THAT AN EMERGENCY TROLLEY/CRASH CART IS IN PLACE BEFORE YOU START

Many medicines regulatory authorities (MRAs) have very specific requirements regarding the contents, checking, and recording of the emergency trolley. The emergency trolley checklist may need to be submitted with all clinical trial applications to the MRA for all trial phases.

The content on the top of the trolley (oxygen tank, automated external defibrillator (AED), suction equipment, cardiopulmonary resuscitation (CPR) algorithms, and stethoscope) is checked every day, and twice a day during participant in-house stays in early phase trials. The rest of the trolley containing emergency drugs and equipment is checked once a month by two appropriately trained staff members (usually the research nurse and pharmacist, or two research nurses). When drugs and/or stock are used from the emergency trolley, it is replaced; the trolley is checked and sealed again.

All trial sites should be aware of their local hospital/regulatory requirements regarding the emergency trolley.

Appendix 7.8 illustrates an example of an emergency trolley checklist showing how the items will be marked. This is not the full list but just an example of what it looks like. Items written in red ink mean it will be expiring at the end of the current month. See comment regarding stock ordered next to it.

COMPILE A WEEKLY UPDATED STATUS REPORT

A weekly status report is an excellent system for updating stakeholders, addressing any concerns of the sponsor/monitor and to get support that you may need to finish the trial successfully (Appendix 7.9).

Here is what the sponsor is concerned about:

- Does this project manager have control of what is happening on the project?
- Does he/she know about any problems or will he/she be surprised down the road?
- Where are we today and are we on track to meet the timelines and recruitment target?

The sponsor is primarily interested in learning if the project will finish on time and within budget. If the news is good, it will relieve their concerns. If the news about the completion date is bad, you will come across as being very frank and forthright about the problems. Then you can immediately address solutions.

You should identify the following:

- The tasks that are causing delays.
- What will happen to the completion date and cost if we do not fix them.
- What you can do about those tasks and delays.
- What the results will be after your corrective action.

Appendix 7.9 is an example of a summary of the study trial and important milestone dates. Updating and forwarding it to your monitor and the relevant team members every week keeps them informed and it is an easy way to measure the progress of the trial. Some contracted research organization (CRO) companies will have their own templates that they prefer, but the basic information normally stays the same. This document is also important for your own site's metrics, and can be used when you update your history of clinical trials at your site. It is a good idea to have the Status Report, the Study Calendar, and the Prestudy Checklist as three spreadsheets in an excel document.

Keypoints
- Detailed planning in advance will identify possible risks and allow time for finding solutions to avoid possible safety issues and violations.
- Communication between the team members is vital and team meetings are essential.
- Identify team members and their responsibilities (Appendix 7.3).
- Monitor progress of planning prior to the start of the trial (Appendix 7.3).
- Use a calendar to plan your study visit dates (Appendix 7.4).
- Prepare a cost estimate/budget to share with your finance department (Appendix 7.5).
- Keep track of your planning with regular updates (Appendix 7.9).
- Have an emergency trolley/crash cart checklist available for inspection (Appendix 7.8).
- Send regular status updates to CRO and study team (Appendix 7.9).
- Remember: "If you fail to plan, you plan to fail."

FURTHER READING

Clinical Research Centre—Spreadsheets. www.crc.uct.ac.za.

APPENDIX 7.1   CASE STUDY

Brief:

"A single center, double blind, randomized, placebo-controlled Phase I study to investigate the safety, tolerability, and pharmacokinetic profile of ascending doses of CRC001 in healthy adult male volunteers."

Synopsis:

The study will evaluate the safety, tolerability, and pharmacokinetic properties of escalating single doses of CRC001 when administered to healthy male volunteers.

Primary objectives:

- To investigate the safety and tolerability of CRC001 when administered to healthy participants.
- To describe the pharmacokinetics of CRC001 in healthy participants after single dose administration.

Secondary objectives:

- To characterize metabolites of CRC001 present in human plasma.
- To determine efficacy of CRC001.

Note: This case study will be used throughout the remaining chapters.

Study Design:

Single center, double blind, randomized, placebo-controlled, ascending dose study.

Study will comprise of 48 healthy male volunteers between the ages of 18 and 55 years.

Study will comprise of up to six cohorts (eight participants in each) that will receive a single, ascending dose (SAD) of CRC001 to assess its safety, tolerability, and pharmacokinetic profile. The starting dose will be 5 mg.

The data obtained from each cohort will undergo a formal review by the Safety Review Team (SRT).

Sample Size:

Up to 48 participants will be enrolled.

Study Duration:

Approximately 58 days for each participant, including a screening period of up to 28 days.

Inclusion Criteria:

1. The subject has completed the written informed consent process.
2. Male participants aged 18–55 years, in good health as determined by past medical history, physical examination, vital signs, electrocardiogram, and laboratory tests at screening.
3. Hematology, clinical chemistry, and urinalysis results at screening that are within the local laboratory reference range or, if outside the range, not clinically significant as judged by the investigator and confirmed and agreed upon by the medical monitor.
4. Body weight of at least 50 kg and a body mass index within the range of 18–32 kg/m^2.
5. Good peripheral venous access.
6. An ability to communicate well with the investigator, to understand and comply with the requirements of the study.
7. Agree to stay in contact with the study site for the duration of the study, provide updated contact information as necessary, and have no current plans to move away from the study area for the duration of the study.

(Continued)

(Continued)

Exclusion Criteria:

1. Any acute illness upon admission to the unit on Day 1 or prior to dosing on Day 1.
2. Use of any other investigational drug within 30 days or five half-lives (whichever is longer) prior to the first dose of CRC001.
3. A history of hypersensitivity to any drugs.
4. A history of anaphylaxis or severe allergic reaction.
5. Resting vital signs (measured 5 minutes in the supine position) at either screening or baseline outside normal ranges as determined by Investigator.
6. A history of clinically significant ECG abnormalities, or ECG abnormalities at either screening or baseline not clinically significant as judged by the investigator.
7. History of malignancy of any organ system (other than localized basal cell carcinoma of the skin), treated or untreated, within the past 5 years.
8. Fertile males defined as all males physiologically capable of conceiving offspring UNLESS the participant agrees to use condoms and ensure that his partner(s) is either not of child-bearing potential or uses a highly effective method of contraception for the entire duration of the study and for 12 weeks following the last study drug administration.
9. Smokers (use of tobacco products) in the previous 3 months.
10. Use of any prescription drugs, herbal supplements, over-the-counter medication or dietary supplements (vitamins included) within 4 weeks prior to initial dosing.
11. Intake of grapefruit or grapefruit juice or other products containing grapefruit within 28 days of the first drug administration of the study drug.
12. Excessive intake of caffeine drinks or energy drinks within 48 hours before admission defined as more than three 250 mL cups, equivalent to roughly 250 mg of caffeine.
13. Donation or loss of 400 mL or more of blood within 8 weeks prior to screening or dosing.
14. Plasma donation (>100 mL) within 60 days prior to dosing.
15. A history of immunodeficiency diseases, including a confirmed positive HIV test result.
16. A positive Hepatitis B surface antigen (HbsAG) or Hepatitis C antibody test result.
17. A history of drug or alcohol abuse within the 12 months prior to dosing, or evidence of such abuse as indicated by the tests and laboratory assays conducted during screening and/or baseline.
18. Any clinically significant mental disorder that could limit the validity of informed consent or the volunteer's ability to comply with protocol requirements.

APPENDIX 7.2 SCHEDULE OF EVENTS

Study Phase	Screening	Baseline	Treatment and Follow-up																		Study End
Visit Numbers	1	2	3												4	5	6	7	8	9	10
Study Days	Day -28 to -2	Day -1	Day 1										2	3	5	7	10	14	19	26	29
Time (h)		-24	Pre dose	0	0.5	1	2	3	4	6	8	12	24	48	96	144	216	312	432	600	672
Informed Consent	x																				
Admission to Center		x																			
Meal record[a]		x — — — — — —	→																		
Inclusion/Exclusion Criteria	x	x	x																		
Medical History	x	x																			
Demography	x																				
Physical Examination	x	x[b]	x[b]											x[b]		x[b]	x[b]		x[b]	x[b]	x[b]
Hepatitis B, C & HIV screen	x																				
Alcohol test, drug screen & serum cotinine	x	x																			
Endocrinology assessments (males)	x	x	x													x		x			
Body Height	x																				
Body Weight	x	x													x	x	x	x			x
Body Temperature	x	x											x		x	x	x	x	x	x	x
Blood Pressure and Heart Rate	x[c]	x	x	x	x	x	x	x	x	x	x	x	x	x	x	x	x	x	x	x	x

ECG	x	x		x	x	x	x	x	x	x	x	x	
Safety Haematology & Biochemistry	x	x	x[c]						x	x	x	x	x
Urinalysis (Dipstick)	x	x	x						x	x		x	x
Study Drug Administration				x									
PK Blood Collection		x	x	x	x	x	x	x	x	x	x	x	x
Pharmacogenetics[d]			x									x	x
Discharge from Centre									x				
Adverse Events	As required												
Serious Adverse Events	As required to 30 days post study completion												
Concomitant Medication / Therapies	x	x	x	As required									

[a] Meal records will be collected for the duration of admission viz., Day -1 to Day 3
[b] Abbreviated (symptom directed) physical exam only to be conducted as relevant
[c] Pre-dose fasting glucose only
[d] Pharmacogenetic sample optional, collected from consented participants ONLY

APPENDIX 7.3 PRESTUDY CHECKLIST

Protocol Number

	Action	Responsible Person	Due Date	Done
1	MCC approval	Regulatory staff	July 31, 2015	√
2	Start-up Meeting (SUM)	Sponsor/CRO	May 16, 2015	√
3	Ethics	Regulatory staff	July 31, 2015	√
4	Check for sufficient steel cabinets for source and site files	Coordinator	July 16, 2015	
5	Check ECG instrument, Dynamap, Holter ECG, alcohol breathalyzer, electronic scale, and calibration certificates	Coordinator	July 16, 2015	
6	Organize caterer	Coordinator	July 16, 2015	
7	Check Internet access	Coordinator	July 16, 2015	
8	Check Sharps and Medical waste	Coordinator	July 16, 2015	
9	Check Photostat machine and paper	Clinical Trial Assistant	July 16, 2015	
10	Check Process laboratory: Centrifuge/freezer/calibration/IATA training	Project Manager	July 16, 2015	
11	Confirm that Financial Contract/Supplier Contracts signed?	Project Manager	August 7, 2015	
12	Review hardcopy of e-CRF or paper CRF	Project Manager	August 7, 2015	
13	Design Source Documents (see source document template)	Project Manager	August 12, 2015	
14	Staff Planning and booking (see staff work schedule)	Coordinator	August 12, 2015	
15	Enrollment plan (see calendar sheet)	Project Manager	August 12, 2015	
16	Book admission ward	Coordinator	August 12, 2015	
17	Site Initiation Meeting (SIM)	CRO/Site	August 19, 2015	
18	Site Files—Check Index vs content (IP source, SAE, and SUSAR)	Project Manager	August 20, 2015	
19	Place Ethics approved newspaper advertisements	Recruiter	August 20, 2015	
20	Prescreen potential participants, contact and book appointments for screening	Recruiter	August 24—ongoing	
21	Database sifting for potential participants/prescreen checklist	Recruiter	August 24—ongoing	
22	Safety Laboratory Kits	Coordinator	As per manual instructions	
23	Source docs review and finalization as well as checklists	Project Manager	1 week prior to screen date	

(Continued)

(Continued)

Protocol Number Action	Responsible Person	Due Date	Done
24 Study supplies and consumables, i.e., Laboratory Kits and manuals. Couriers, Import and Export permits, waybills	Coordinator/ Laboratory Assistant	Ongoing	
25 Order more laboratory visit kits when necessary	Coordinator/ Laboratory Assistant	Ongoing	
26 Medical consumables (i.e., webcol swabs, cannulas, cotton balls, etc.)	Clinical Trial Assistant	3 weeks prior to first screen date	
27 Check that Ice available	Laboratory Assistant	Day prior to needed	
28 Prepare for Screening: participant folders, ward, checklists	Coordinator/ CTA	1 day prior to planned screening	
29 Meals—confirm with caterer	Coordinator	1 week prior to admission	
30 Participant reimbursement	CTA	Ongoing	

APPENDIX 7.4   STUDY CALENDAR

Date	Cohort 1	Cohort 2	Cohort 3	Cohort 4	Cohort 5	Cohort 6
	Wed	**Screen Visit**				
May 01, 2016	Thu	**Screen Visit**				
May 02, 2016	Fri	**Screen Visit**				
May 03, 2016	Sat	Day −10				
May 04, 2016	Sun	Day −9				
May 05, 2016	Mon	Day −8	**Screen Visit**			
May 06, 2016	Tue	Day −7	**Screen Visit**			
May 07, 2016	Wed	Day −6	**Screen Visit**			
May 08, 2016	Thu	Day −5	Day −19			
May 09, 2016	Fri	Day −4	Day −18			
May 10, 2016	Sat	Day −3	Day −17			
May 11, 2016	Sun	Day −2	Day −16			

(Continued)

Date	Cohort 1	Cohort 2	Cohort 3	Cohort 4	Cohort 5	Cohort 6
May 12, 2016	Mon	**Day − 1 Admit**	Day −15			
May 13, 2016	Tue	**Day 1— Random**	Day −14			
May 14, 2016	Wed	**Day 2**	Day −13			
May 15, 2016	Thu	**Day 3 Discharge**	Day −12			
May 16, 2016	Fri	Day 4	Day −11	**Screen Visit**		
May 17, 2016	Sat	**Day 5**	Day −10			
May 18, 2016	Sun	Day 6	Day −9			
May 19, 2016	Mon	**Day 7**	Day −8			
May 20, 2016	Tue	Day 8	Day −7	**Screen Visit**	Day −28	
May 21, 2016	Wed	Day 9	Day −6	**Screen Visit**	Day −27	
May 22, 2016	Thu	**Day 10**	Day −5	Day −12	**Screen Visit**	
May 23, 2016	Fri	Day 11	Day −4	Day −11	**Screen Visit**	
May 24, 2016	Sat	Day 12	Day −3	Day −10	Day −24	
May 25, 2016	Sun	Day 13	Day −2	Day −9	Day −23	
May 26, 2016	Mon	**Day 14**	**Day − 1 Admit**	Day −8	Day −22	
May 27, 2016	Tue	Day 15	**Day 1 - Random**	Day −7	Day −21	
May 28, 2016	Wed	Day 16	**Day 2**	Day −6	Day −20	
May 29, 2016	Thu	Day 17	**Day 3 Discharge**	Day −5	Day −19	
May 30, 2016	Fri	Day 18	Day 4	Day −4	**Screen Visit**	
May 31, 2016	Sat	**Day 19**	**Day 5**	Day −3	Day −17	
June 01, 2016	Sun	Day 20	Day 6	Day −2	Day −16	
June 02, 2016	Mon	Day 21	**Day 7**	**Day − 1 Admit**	Day −15	
June 03, 2016	Tue	Day 22	Day 8	**Day 1— Random**	Day −14	
June 04, 2016	Wed	Day 23	Day 9	**Day 2**	Day −13	
June 05, 2016	Thu	Day 24	**Day 10**	**Day 3 Discharge**	Day −12	

(*Continued*)

(Continued)

Date	Cohort 1	Cohort 2	Cohort 3	Cohort 4	Cohort 5	Cohort 6
June 06, 2016	Fri	Day 25	Day 11	Day 4	Day −11	
June 07, 2016	Sat	**Day 26**	Day 12	**Day 5**	Day −10	
June 08, 2016	Sun	Day 27	Day 13	Day 6	Day −9	
June 09, 2016	Mon	Day 28	**Day 14**	**Day 7**	Day −8	
June 10, 2016	Tue	**Day 29**	Day 15	Day 8	Day −7	**Screen Visit**
June 11, 2016	Wed		Day 16	Day 9	Day −6	**Screen Visit**
June 12, 2016	Thu		Day 17	**Day 10**	Day −5	**Screen Visit**
June 13, 2016	Fri		Day 18	Day 11	Day −4	Day −13
June 14, 2016	Sat		**Day 19**	Day 12	Day −3	Day −12
June 15, 2016	Sun		Day 20	Day 13	Day −2	Day −11
June 16, 2016	Mon		Day 21	**Day 14**	**Day − 1 Admit**	Day −10
June 17, 2016	Tue		Day 22	Day 15	**Day 1— Random**	Day −9
June 18, 2016	Mon		Day 23	Day 16	**Day 2**	Day −8
June 19, 2016	Tue		Day 24	Day 17	**Day 3 Discharge**	Day −7
June 20, 2016	Wed		Day 25	Day 18	Day 4	Day −6
June 21, 2016	Thu		**Day 26**	**Day 19**	Day 5	Day −5
June 22, 2016	Fri		Day 27	Day 20	Day 6	Day −4
June 23, 2016	Sat		Day 28	Day 21	**Day 7**	Day −3
June 24, 2016	Sun		**Day 29**	Day 22	Day 8	Day −2
June 25, 2016	Mon			Day 23	Day 9	**Day − 1 Admit**
June 26, 2016	Tue			Day 24	**Day 10**	**Day 1— Random**
June 27, 2016	Wed			Day 25	Day 11	**Day 2**
June 28, 2016	Thu			**Day 26**	Day 12	**Day 3 Discharge**

The bold usage of words indicate the actual study visits.

APPENDIX 7.5 STUDY BUDGET

STUDY TITLE:					
Sponsor :					
Study Code:					
Principal Investigator:					

Number of patients screened:	96		Number of patients randomized:		48
Recruitment rate/month:	2:1		Number of visits:		9
Study closing date:	Feb-15				

TEAM MEMBERS	FUNCTION		Cost per unit per hour	Units to be used (total hours of work)	BUDGET (cost x total hours)
COSTS - PER PATIENT:					Total hours
	PI		R 1	20	R 20
	Lead Investigator		R 1	40	R 40
	Project Manager		R 1	32	R 32
	Study Coordinator		R 1	40	R 40
	Research Nurses x (day)		R 1	60	R 60
	Research Nurses x (night)		R 1	60	R 60
	Lab assistant x (day)		R 1	60	R 60
	Research pharmacist (dispensing/patient)		R 1	60	R 60
	Data Base Designer (Paper CRF)		R 1		R 0
	Data Base Designer (e-CRF)		R 1		R 0
	Data Capturing		R 1	10	R 10
	Query resolution, data base lock		R 1	4	R 4
	Safety Report template, Data management protocol		R 1		R 0
	Compile draft safety report		R 1		R 0
		Sub total:			R386
CONSUMABLES:					
Stationery			R 1	1	R 1
Photocopying (per page)			R 1	1	R 1
Medical & ward			R 1	1	R 1
		Sub total:			R 3
ACCOMMODATION /VENUE REQUIREMENTS:					
Accommodation					
Ward/Consulting Rooms:	Screen: pts per day over x days		R 1	1	R 1
	Treatment: x night stay over		R 1	1	R 1
Meals	Snacks (per person) x snacks x pts		R 1	1	R 1
	Meals (per Person) x meals x pts		R 1	1	R 1
		Sub total:			R 4
		Total Costs Per Patient:			R 393
SITE COSTS:					
Protocol Development (consulting fee)			R 1	10	R 10
	PI Protocol & ICD design		R 1	40	R 40
	PM - protocol & ICD design		R 1	20	R 20
Finance Mx (incl Budget development)			R 1	20	R 20

REGULATORY SUBMISSIONS:				
Regulatory officer		R 1	40	R 40
MCC submission		R 1	1	R 1
Ethics submission		R 1	1	R 1
RESOURCES:				
Safety Labs (Haem, Chem, Urinalysis, DOA)		R 1	1	R 1
IATA Training	3 x staff @ R1 per staff member	R 1	4	R 4
GCP training	4 x refresher course @ R1 per staff member	R 1	4	R 4
	4 x starter course @ R1 per staff member	R 1	4	R 4
Pharmacy:	Pharmacy start-up costs	R 1	1	R 1
	Fridge and probe for IMP storage	R 1	1	R 1
	IMP destruction*	R 1	1	R 1
*only charged if site is required to dispose of IMP				
Archiving	Archiving	R 1	1	R 1
Admin start-up Fee		R 1	1	R 1
Sub total:				R 150
PROJECT MANAGEMENT:				
Advertising	Local newspapers (x newspapers x weeks)	R 1	1	R 1
Sub total:				R 1
Total Site Costs:				R151
PER PATIENT COSTS + TOTAL SITE COSTS:				R 544
OVERHEAD COSTS AT 20%				R109
GRAND TOTAL:				R 653

APPENDIX 7.6   STAFF WORK SCHEDULE

27 May 2014: Day 1 (Dosing)								
	1	**2**	**3**	**4**	**5**	**6**	**7**	**8**
Check crashcart, check ECG paper & synchronize time, hand warmers, Freezer temp				5:00				
Ablutions/urine/offer water to drink				5:30				
Remove water from bedside	6:00	6:08	6:16	6:24	6:32	6:40	6:48	6:56
Med hx/PE (abbrev)	6:40	6:45	6:50	6:55	7:00	7:05	7:10	7:15
Start rest	6:55	7:03	7:11	7:19	7:27	7:35	7:43	7:51
BP/HR/Temp (hand warmer)	7:00	7:08	7:16	7:24	7:32	7:40	7:48	7:56
ECG	7:02	7:10	7:18	7:26	7:34	7:42	7:50	7:58
ELIGIBILITY	7:04	7:12	7:20	7:28	7:36	7:44	7:52	8:00
Cannulate	7:10	7:18	7:26	7:34	7:42	7:50	7:58	8:06
Ice cups at bed	7:35	7:43	7:51	7:59	8:07	8:15	8:23	8:31
PK 00 (pre-dose) Safety bloods/PG sample/sit up	**7:40**	**7:48**	**7:56**	**8:04**	**8:12**	**8:20**	**8:28**	**8:36**
Phone pharmacy	8:10	8:18	8:26	8:34	8:42	8:50	8:58	9:06
Dose/lie semi-recumbant	**8:30**	**8:38**	**8:46**	**8:54**	**9:02**	**9:10**	**9:18**	**9:26**
QC of source up to dosing				8:00 - 9:00				
Rest (supine)	8:50	8:58	9:06	9:14	9:22	9:30	9:38	9:46
Hand warmer	8:50	8:58	9:06	9:14	9:22	9:30	9:38	9:46
Ice cups at bed	8:55	9:03	9:11	9:19	9:27	9:35	9:43	9:51
BP/HR	8:55	9:03	9:11	9:19	9:27	9:35	9:43	9:51
PK 01 (0.5 hr)	**9:00**	**9:08**	**9:16**	**9:24**	**9:32**	**9:40**	**9:48**	**9:56**
Start rest/hand warmer	9:15	9:23	9:31	9:39	9:47	9:55	10:03	10:11
BP/HR/Temp	9:20	9:28	9:36	9:44	9:52	10:00	10:08	10:16
Ice cups at bed	9:20	9:28	9:36	9:44	9:52	10:00	10:08	10:16
ECG	9:25	9:33	9:41	9:49	9:57	10:05	10:13	10:21
PK 02 (1 hr)	**9:30**	**9:38**	**9:46**	**9:54**	**10:02**	**10:10**	**10:18**	**10:26**
Start rest/hand warmer	10:15	10:23	10:31	10:39	10:47	10:55	11:03	11:11
BP/HR	10:20	10:28	10:36	10:44	10:52	11:00	11:08	11:16
Ice cups at bed	10:20	10:28	10:36	10:44	10:52	11:00	11:08	11:16
ECG	10:25	10:33	10:41	10:49	10:57	11:05	11:13	11:21
PK 03 (2 hr)	**10:30**	**10:38**	**10:46**	**10:54**	**11:02**	**11:10**	**11:18**	**11:26**
Water may be taken	10:30	10:38	10:46	10:54	11:02	11:10	11:18	11:26
Start rest	11:15	11:23	11:31	11:39	11:47	11:55	12:03	12:11
BP/HR	11:20	11:28	11:36	11:44	11:52	12:00	12:08	12:16
Ice cups at bed	11:20	11:28	11:36	11:44	11:52	12:00	12:08	12:16
ECG	11:25	11:33	11:41	11:49	11:57	12:05	12:13	12:21

PK 04 (3 hr)	11:30	11:38	11:46	11:54	12:02	12:10	12:18	12:26
Start rest	12:15	12:23	12:31	12:39	12:47	12:55	13:03	13:11
BP/HR/Temp	12:20	12:28	12:36	12:44	12:52	13:00	13:08	13:16
Ice cups at bed	12:20	12:28	12:36	12:44	12:52	13:00	13:08	13:16
ECG	12:25	12:33	12:41	12:49	12:57	13:05	13:13	13:21
PK 05 (4 hr)	12:30	12:38	12:46	12:54	13:02	13:10	13:18	13:26
Lunch meal record	13:00	13:08	13:16	13:24	13:32	13:40	13:48	13:56
Change stillette in canula	13:30	13:38	13:46	13:54	14:02	14:10	14:18	14:26
QC of source	13:00–15:00							
Start rest/hand warmer	14:15	14:23	14:31	14:39	14:47	14:55	15:03	15:11
BP/HR	14:20	14:28	14:36	14:44	14:52	15:00	15:08	15:16
Ice cups at bed	14:20	14:28	14:36	14:44	14:52	15:00	15:08	15:16
ECG	14:25	14:33	14:41	14:49	14:57	15:05	15:13	15:21
PK 06 (6 hr)	14:30	14:38	14:46	14:54	15:02	15:10	15:18	15:26
Change stillette in canula	15:30	15:38	15:46	15:54	16:02	16:10	16:18	16:26
Snack meal record	16:00	16:08	16:16	16:24	16:32	16:40	16:48	16:56
Start rest/hand warmer	16:15	16:23	16:31	16:39	16:47	16:55	17:03	17:11
BP/HR	16:20	16:28	16:36	16:44	16:52	17:00	17:08	17:16
Ice cups at bed	16:20	16:28	16:36	16:44	16:52	17:00	17:08	17:16
PK 07 (8 hr)	16:30	16:38	16:46	16:54	17:02	17:10	17:18	17:26
Check crashcart & emergency bells	17h30							
Change stillette in canula	17:45	17:53	18:01	18:09	18:17	18:25	18:33	18:41
Dinner meal record	18:00	18:08	18:16	18:24	18:32	18:40	18:48	18:56
Handover to night staff	18:00							
Change stillette in canula	19:30							
Hand warmer	20:10	20:18	20:26	20:34	20:42	20:50	20:58	21:06
Ice cups at bed & rest	20:22	20:30	20:38	20:46	20:54	21:02	21:10	21:18
BP/HR	20:27	20:35	20:43	20:51	20:59	21:07	21:15	21:23
PK 08 (12 hr)	20:30	20:38	20:46	20:54	21:02	21:10	21:18	21:26
Snack meal record	20:45	20:53	21:01	21:09	21:17	21:25	21:33	21:41
Nil per mouth	22:00	22:08	22:16	22:24	22:32	22:40	22:48	22:56

Staff Colour Coding:

Investigator	Nurse 1	Nurse 2	Nurse 3			Night	Data Capturer

Assistant	

APPENDIX 7.7 STOCK LIST

	Clinical Research Centre			CRC 4.1 Stock Checklist	
Trial No.			**Sponsor:**		

Details of stock take:

Stock type*	Description (*Examples*)	No.	Expiry	Order	Comment
	Alcohol swabs				
	Cotton gauze				
	Cotton wool balls				
	G20 Cannulas				
	Latex gloves - large				
	Latex gloves - medium				
	Latex gloves - small				
	Linen savers				
	Micropore				
	Laboratory Kits				
	Syringes – 10 ml				
	Syringes – 5 ml				
	Thermometers				
	Tourniquets				
	ECG electrodes				
	Scissors				

*Stock type:
MC, Med cons.
ET, Emergency trolley
WG, Ward gen.
C , Catering
O, Other (detail)

Completed by	Designation	Signature	Date

APPENDIX 7.8   EMERGENCY TROLLEY CHECKLIST

Emergency Trolley Checklist

Ward: _____   Month: _____

DESCRIPTION: _____

Top Shelf of Trolley (to be checked every day when participants in ward)

Days of month			1	2	3	4	5	6	7	8	9	10	11	12	13	14	15	16	17	18	19	20	21	22	23	24	25	26	27	28	29	30	31
Oxygen Cylinder 0.47Kg with Tubing and regulator (pin index)	4 Oct 2014	1																															
Automated External Defibrillator (AED)	N/A	1																															
Adult Multifunction Electrode Pads	Nov 2014	1 pair																															
Drip stand	N/A	1																															
Latest AHS resuscitation algorithms	N/A	N/A																															
Dash 6000 Cardiac Monitor	N/A	1																															
Battery portable suction (with cord)	N/A	1																															
Suction Catheter Size 14	N/A	1																															
Yankauer Suction	N/A	1																															
Stethoscope	N/A	1																															
Mask (40%) with Tubing	N/A	1																															
Bag Valve Mask Reservoir & masks		1																															
Transfer Letter		1																															
AM Checked by: (Initial & Date)																																	
PM Checked by: (Initial & Date)																																	

Top Left Shelf (to be checked once a month or after use)

DRUGS:	Expiry date	Amount	
Amiotach / Amiodarone	May 2016	5	
Adrenaline 1:1000 (1mg/1ml)	20xOct2016	20	
Atropine 1.0 mg/ 1ml	Dec 2016	10	
Calcium Chloride	March 2017	5	
Dextrose in water 50%(20ml)	Feb 2017	10	
Dextrose in water 50%(20ml)	Jul 2015	2	
Furosemide / Lasix 20mg/2ml	Jun 2015	5	
Ipratropium bromide/ Atrovent (0,5mg/2ml)	Jun 2015	4	
Lignocaine 2%	2xOct 2018 4xSep2019	2	
Magnesium Sulphate 1g / 2ml	June 2015	5	
Nitrolingual Spray 0,4mg /spray	Jan 2017	1	
Potassium Chloride	Oct 2016	2	
Promethazine / Phenergan 25mg	2xApr 2017 3xMay2017	5	
SoluCortef 100mg/2ml	March 2017	5	
SoluCortef 100mg/2ml	Oct 2015	1	
Sodium Chloride 0,9% 10ml	Feb 2016	10	
Sterile water 10ml	Sep 2015	20	
Ventolin / Albuterol Salbutamol (5,0mg/2.5ml)	May 2015	5	
Disprin 300mg	Feb2016	8	
Ativan injection / Lorazepam 4mg/1ml (stored in Lab Fridge)	Dec2015	10	
NovaRapid 10 ml (stored in Lab Fridge)	May 2015	1	
GlucaGen Hypokit (stored in Lab Fridge)	Mar 2015	2	Ordered 22 Feb 2015

APPENDIX 7.9   STATUS REPORT

Study:						Date & Initial:	04 Feb 15 / Coordinator		
Contracted No. of Participants:	48					Principal Investigator:	Prof ABC		

Screening:	*FSFSCR = 1st subject 1st screen date		*FSFE = 1st subject 1st dosing date		*FSLV = 1st subject last visit date (SFU)	*LSLE = Last subject 1st dosing date	*LSLV = Last subject last Follow-up proc
Dates:	30-Apr-14		13-May-14		10-Jun-14	18-Nov-14	02-Feb-15

Actual dates not planned dates

	Chrt 1	Chrt 2	Chrt 3	Chrt 4	Chrt 5	Chrt 6	Total:	Comment
Pre-screened:	50	123	78	102	136	95	**584**	*You can add comments every week regarding recruitment difficulties, strategy etc.*
Booked for Screen:	30	28	30	27	30	30	**175**	
Screened:	20	16	14	22	17	15	**104**	
Screen failures:	12	8	6	14	9	7	**56**	
Ready to Enroll:	8	8	8	8	8	8	**48**	
Randomized:	8	8	8	8	8	8	**48**	
R withd/drop outs:								
Ongoing:							**0**	
Study Completed:	8	8	8	8	8	8	**48**	

Chapter 8

Recruitment and Retention

Brenda Wright

Chapter Outline

RECRUITMENT

ICH-GCP E6 Section 4.2.1 mentions that "the investigator should be able to demonstrate (e.g. based on retrospective data) a potential for recruiting the required number of suitable subjects within the agreed recruitment period."

This places a lot of pressure on the investigator and the site, and if you have not planned in advance, you may very well run into trouble with agreed timelines. The secret is to realize what motivates participants to be part of a clinical trial, the reasons why some participants will not join, and to identify your recruitment challenges before you start and during the screening process.

Motivations for Participating in a Clinical Trial

1. Access to services such as medical care, medication, investigators/doctors, specialists, and regular follow-ups play a big role in patient trials.
2. Emotions and social motivations—participants develop a sense of belonging. They enjoy the comfort of the facilities. Some sees it as a social outing. Participants have trust in the staff and facility.
3. Other motivations include their ability to contribute to scientific progress and the opportunity to learn more about their own illness/disease.

A Comprehensive and Practical Guide to Clinical Trials.
DOI: http://dx.doi.org/10.1016/B978-0-12-804729-3.00008-0

4. Remuneration—Even though the ethics behind remuneration is very sensitive, it is a motivating factor for participants (especially healthy participants). The participants do not want to be "out of pocket" and their traveling costs and time off work should be remunerated.

Why Participants Will not Join

1. There is still a perception that participants are "guinea pigs."
2. In some countries the research industry has a very poor reputation.
3. Participants are fearful of possible side effects.
4. Participants on the placebo arm may have concerns regarding nontreatment.
5. The complexity of treatment may deter potential participants.
6. Alternative, satisfactory treatment may be available already.
7. Negative press releases have a big influence on recruitment for clinical trials.

Recruitment Challenges

Now that we understand why a participant will want to be part of a clinical trial or not, we can assess other recruitment challenges with which we are faced.

1. *Protocol review and recruitment*: When a site/investigator look at a protocol synopsis and/or the protocol, it is important to recognize possible recruitment challenges before committing to the project. What do we look at when reviewing the protocol from a recruitment perspective?
    i. Note the specific patient population required. Do you have access to this population?
    ii. Protocol inclusion/exclusion criteria and complexity of trial: Will your participant database and other recruitment methods be sufficient to fit this criteria?
    iii. Check the recruitment target expected from you. Is this viable? How many participants will you be able to recruit per week/month?
    iv. The duration of the study and the frequency of the visits can play a huge role in your recruitment success as well as retention of participants until the end of the trial. Ensure that it is feasible for your site and the participant population you are looking at.
    v. Calculate the amount of hours/labor the trial will require. Do you have the time and do you have a sufficient support structure (facilities and staff) to conduct the trial successfully?
2. *Trial site*
    i. Do you have competing studies running at the moment and if so will your patient database be large enough to recruit for all competing trials?
    ii. Do you have adequately trained staff to support you?

3. *Participant issues*
    i. Literacy and informed consent. Will you need translators, parents/ legal guardians, and/or an independent witness to sign the informed consent document?
    ii. Participant commitment. Ensure that the participant, carers, and legal guardians understand the commitment required to participate in a clinical trial.
    iii. Participant perception. Participants must have a clear understanding of what will be expected from them during the whole process.
    iv. Be aware of possible pressure from social and/or culture circles regarding participation in a clinical trial.
4. *Regulatory body approvals*

    In certain countries the regulatory approvals can take between 3 and 6 months. Make sure that you take this into consideration when you commit to timelines, as a delayed approval can cut into your recruitment time. Chapter 4, Regulatory Requirements, includes details of requirements for several countries.

Recruitment Options

There are various options/ways recruitment can be done. The options you choose are directly related to your clinical trial and participant population. Ensure that you have your recruitment strategy in place prior to budget negotiations so as not to omit advertising costs, etc., from your budget. Examples of some options are:

1. participant pool/database,
2. referral from other physicians,
3. site and/or hospital databases and archives,
4. community outreach groups,
5. patient support groups,
6. public speaking engagements,
7. health care centers and institutions,
8. advertising—this can be in the form of:
    i. centralized campaigns,
    ii. site generated advertisements,
    iii. Internet usage/social media,
    iv. media (TV, Radio, Flyers, Newspapers),
    v. Remember that your advertising materials must be approved by your local Ethics committee and should not include Sponsor names.

Achieving Recruitment Targets

1. Set recruitment targets for available dates. Start recruitment on target date. Do not delay. Keep track of your target, and try not to fall behind.

2. Use recruitment logs to track your progress and determine the reasons should you fall behind.
3. Adapt your strategy to increase recruitment numbers.
4. Be flexible in your approach.
5. Have regular feedback meetings with your recruitment staff.

RETENTION

Reaching your recruitment target is always a great relief, but that is only half the battle won. The next challenge is participant retention.

There are three main reasons why participant retention is very important:

1. You will be under contractual obligation. The Clinical Trial Agreement would normally state the number of participants expected to complete the trial.
2. The Clinical Trial Agreement may also dictate the financial impact if participants do not complete the trial.
3. The most important reason: the success of your trial may depend on the number of participants completing the trial.

Signs of Potential Nonadherence

1. Participant starts missing visits.
2. It becomes difficult to reach participant by phone and participant does not return calls.
3. Participant starts complaining about the site visits (too long, etc.).
4. Participant shows signs of impatience during his/her visit.

Reasons for Resistance

1. Adverse Events (AE)—participant may be worried about the risk to himself.
2. Participant may have transport problems (especially in countries where public transport is not easily accessible or expensive).
3. The caregiver that has to accompany participant is too busy.
4. The participant may experience problems with his/her employer regarding time off to attend trial visits.
5. Participant may be relocated to another city.

If you are able to detect these signs early on, you may be able to address the issue and prevent the participant from nonadherence and withdrawing from the trial before the end.

Useful Tips for Participant Retention

1. Anticipate problems:
   a. Do not recruit "doubtful" participants.
   b. Find out as much as possible about your participant.
   c. Obtain as many contact details as possible: family, friends, caregiver, etc.
2. Make the trial visits "special":
   a. Participant must feel special. Let them know how important they are and emphasize the contribution to society they make.
   b. Be approachable and available.
   c. Ensure that the waiting room is informal and comfortable.
   d. Thank them after each visit and make sure their appointment card is updated for the next visit.
3. Regular contact with the participants:
   a. Keeping regular contact with the participant during the trial builds a relationship between you and the participant.
   b. It assists you in keeping track of where the participant is.
   c. Regular contact will improve compliance.
4. Organize extra visits if necessary.
   Calling a participant back for an unscheduled visit could be for various reasons:
   a. Participant reported an AE and Investigator calls them back to the site for an unscheduled visit. This will make the participant feel cared for and looked after.
   b. Should the participants show noncompliance, it is always beneficial to arrange an unscheduled visit to confirm the reasons and encourage the participant.

Keypoints

Recruitment
- Principal Investigator should be able to demonstrate a potential for recruiting the required number of suitable participants within the agreed recruitment period.
- Identify recruitment challenges in advance and during the recruitment period.
- Understand the participant's motivation to be part of a clinical trial or why they will not participate.
- Recruitment options are directly related to your clinical trial and participant population.
- Set recruitment targets and monitor progress.
- Regular feedback meetings with recruitment staff are essential.

(Continued)

Keypoints (Continued)

Retention

- The success of your trial may depend on the number of participants completing the trial.
- Be aware of signs of potential nonadherence.
- Anticipate problems early on.
- Keep regular contact with your participants.
- Organize extra visits where necessary.

FURTHER READING

ICH-GCP Section 4.2.1.

Chapter 9

Training

Brenda Wright

Chapter Outline

International Council for Harmonization-Good Clinical Practice (ICH-GCP) guidelines state that the Principal Investigator (PI) is the leader of the team who conducts the clinical trial. The PIs are responsible for adequate protocol training of all staff. They may delegate tasks to adequately trained, qualified staff, but they may not delegate responsibility.

The PI does not have to conduct all the training, as most of the training will be done by the Sponsor/CRP, external parties such as the data management company, central laboratories, etc. The PI may delegate the training to trained, qualified staff. Training is an ongoing activity prior to and during the conduct of a trial. All training done for protocol amendments, etc., must be documented as well.

INTERNAL TRAINING

1. Orientation—all new staff to the clinical team should have an orientation program. This program will familiarize staff with the facility (site), policies, HR, access control, confidentiality, etc. The orientation program should be documented and signed by all new staff on completion.
2. Standard operating procedures (SOP)—A typical trial site would have generic SOPs regarding procedures and processes that will cover most trials. In Investigator lead trials, SOPs are usually protocol specific. Some Sponsors and contracted research organization (CRO) companies will also provide their own policies and SOPs for training. Procedures/techniques should be descriptive and where possible demonstrated. SOP training must be completed prior to the start of the clinical trial and signed by all members of the clinical team.

A Comprehensive and Practical Guide to Clinical Trials.
DOI: http://dx.doi.org/10.1016/B978-0-12-804729-3.00009-2

3. Health and Safety—This may be covered in the Quality Management policies/procedures, but can also be covered in SOPs. Part of Health and Safety would be Basic Life Support training and/or Advanced Cardiac Life Support training by external accredited vendors where applicable.

EXTERNAL TRAINING

1. Start-Up (Investigator Meeting)
   a. In Pharmaceutical Trials this meeting is organized and presented by the Sponsor. Where multiple sites are involved, the meeting will be held at a central venue or via web-n-air meetings.
   b. In Investigator lead trials this meeting will be the PI's responsibility and it is often combined with the Site Initiation meeting (SIM).
   c. Start-Up Meetings may be arranged and conducted prior to Regulatory approvals but SIMs should be arranged after regulatory and other approvals are in place.
   d. During this meeting, the study protocol will be discussed in detail.
   e. The PI and study coordinator will be invited to attend this meeting. Should they not be able to attend, the PI may nominate a subinvestigator or pharmacist to attend the meeting with the Sponsor's approval. During this meeting, the CRO and site monitor will also receive training. If this meeting is held via web-n-air, it is beneficial to involve as many of the study team members to attend as possible.
   f. Attending this meeting is vitally important to the study team. This may be the only opportunity the PI and study coordinator have to meet with the Sponsor, central laboratory, data management team, and to identify possible challenges regarding the protocol and conduct of the trial. It also provides the best platform for the representative study team members to ask questions and address any uncertainties regarding the protocol, study procedures, laboratory procedures, data capturing, etc.
   g. Ensure that you are familiar with the content of the protocol prior to the meeting.
   h. External vendors such as the central laboratory, data management team, study-specific specialized equipment (ECG's, Spirometry equipment, electronic diaries, trial slates, etc.) will also attend the meeting and provide training.
   i. Timelines are discussed as well as targets (number of participants to be enrolled) and recruitment strategies.

    j. A certificate of Attendance and a flash-drive and/or a print-out of the meeting presentation slides will be provided to the site team. The certificate of attendance will be filed together with all other training records in the study site file.

2. On-Line Training

    a. Most Pharmaceutical clinical trials also require certain staff members to complete electronic training. Examples of this are Protocol, Investigator Brochure, summary of GCP guidelines, data capturing, investigative medicinal product (IMP) specifications, IVRS/IWRS registration of participant enrollment and laboratory procedures. Records of completion for this training must be kept in the Study Site File as well. This training is role specific and investigators, coordinators, data capturers, pharmacists, etc., will each have certain modules to complete. This training must be completed prior to the start of a clinical trial.

3. Site Initiation Meeting

    a. The SIM is held after all approvals are in place and all study supplies have been delivered.

    b. This meeting is usually chaired by the CRO company/study monitor, but in investigator lead trials, the PI takes on this responsibility.

    c. The meeting is held at the site and so it should be possible for most team members to attend.

    d. During this meeting, the protocol, timelines, recruitment strategy, IMP storage and dosing procedures, data capturing, laboratory procedures and shipment arrangements, and monitoring plan will be discussed.

    e. The monitor will provide the site with the Investigator Site Files and will confirm that all study supplies, source documents, etc., are in place.

    f. The signed attendance register and presentation/minutes will be filed in the study site files.

4. GCP/GLCP and International Air Transport Association (IATA) training

    a. All study staff must have GCP training done by an accredited training facility. Certificates are kept in the site files. In most countries a refresher course must be done every 3 years.

    b. GLCP is the laboratory version of GCP. In some countries this training is sufficient for laboratory staff but in others, GCP training is required as well.

    c. IATA or similar training is required for laboratory staff that is responsible for shipment of biological samples. This training should usually be repeated every 2 years.

Keypoints

- The Principal Investigator is responsible for adequate protocol training of all staff.
- The Principal Investigator may delegate training to suitable, qualified staff.
- Training is ongoing and must always be documented.
- All study staff must be GCP trained.
- Laboratory staff responsible for shipments must have IATA or similar training.

FURTHER READING

ICH-GCP Sections 2.8 and 4.1.

Chapter 10

Data Management

Annemie Stewart

Chapter Outline

The essential elements of Good Data Management Practice from study conception to data lock and archive.

A study is only as good as the data. Good data management ensures that data are of consistently high quality, meet regulatory, legal, and funder requirements, and ensures the security, authenticity, and future availability of the data. This chapter reviews all the key steps to follow throughout the project lifecycle (Fig. 10.1).

A Comprehensive and Practical Guide to Clinical Trials.
DOI: http://dx.doi.org/10.1016/B978-0-12-804729-3.00010-9
© 2017 Elsevier Inc. All rights reserved.

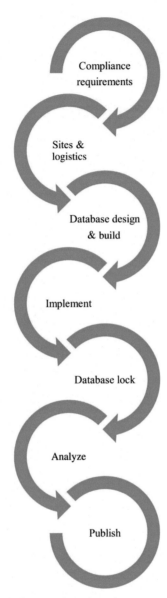

FIGURE 10.1 Key steps to follow throughout the project.

ESTABLISH COMPLIANCE REQUIREMENTS

During the funding application and protocol development stage, find out which rules and regulations will be applicable to the study. This will differ between countries and geographical regions (e.g., the European Union or

EU compared to the United States). Consider and document each of the following types of requirements that may apply to the study.

Legislation and Regulatory Authorities

Drug trials need to take into account the compliance requirements of the country/countries where the study will take place, as well as those of regulatory authorities in foreign markets where the drug may eventually need to be registered (e.g., with the Food and Drug Administration or FDA). These may require the data to be in a specific type of system, format, or data standard (e.g., Clinical Data Acquisition Standards Harmonization or CDASH, Clinical Data Interchange Standards Consortium [1], which is a globally used data format).

Good Clinical Practice/Ethical Considerations

It is always important to adhere to Good Clinical Practice (GCP) and ethical principles. If no locally adapted GCP guidelines exist, the International Council for Harmonisation (ICH)-GCP guidelines should be used, ICH E6 [2]. ICH-GCP covers topics like participant confidentiality and the need to separate identifying information from study data. ICH-GCP also discusses the following data management requirements:

- Data systems must be developed in accordance with the protocol, by suitably qualified individuals.
- Data systems used must be validated, that is, must have been developed and tested according to documented procedures, and have standard operating procedures (SOPs) for their use.
- Data systems must have a tamper-proof audit trail, that is, a time-stamped history of the data captured and changes made to the data, including who captured/changed the data, that cannot be altered directly by anyone.
- Data systems must allow access only to authorized users, which means that the users must be identifiable individual persons whose names appear on a delegation log for data-related tasks on the study.
- Study data must be adequately backed up—preferably in physically distinct locations.
- Data systems must maintain allocation concealment where required by the protocol.

Site-Specific Rules

Sites and investigators may also have to take into account institutional, company, unit, or facility-specific rules about data management. Collect all of these for consideration.

Funder/Sponsor Requirements

The funder and/or sponsor of your study may have their own rules to comply with. Some may even require that particular components of data management be ceded to a particular vendor altogether. The funder and/or sponsor may have specific reporting requirements (e.g., they may require reports indicating the number of subjects enrolled, randomized, completed, etc. in a particular format at particular time intervals during the study) that need to be taken into account during database development. Increasingly funders/sponsors require a data management plan during the funding application and issue guidelines/regulations to this effect. The data management plan summarizes how data are handled throughout the project lifecycle (example available online). The plan usually covers a description of the type of data, how it is generated and collected, how it is documented/curated, data security measures, plans for data sharing, and a list of responsibilities and the responsible persons [3].

Document all the relevant rules and regulations that apply to the study data—this should be kept in the Trial Master File. Where more than one rule applies, the more conservative approach should be selected and the decision documented.

CONSIDER SITES AND LOGISTICS

Source

Source documents are all of the original documents and records of drug trial activities, including measurements and observations of the participants (read Chapter 13, Source Document, for a thorough discussion). While drug trials historically used only paper source documents, technological advances mean that data can sometimes be recorded directly in electronic form. For example, an instrument that measures blood pressure and records this *directly* into the database, completely eliminates the need to first write down the blood pressure on a paper source document, and so reduces the risk of error. Increasingly drug trials have a mix of paper and electronic data sources. Electronic data sources become part of the entire data system, and as such have to be reliable and validated.

Case Report Form

The case report form (CRF) contains all of the data that need to be reported for each trial participant, and should therefore cover all of the stated study objectives including reportable safety data points according to the protocol. Traditionally CRFs were highly structured paper forms completed by study staff at each site (often in duplicate or triplicate) by transcribing information recorded in the source documents. Paper CRFs were then transferred to data capturers who would enter the information into an electronic database. However, as computers and the Internet become more and more accessible to studies, electronic CRFs (eCRFs) are increasing in popularity. Study staff at each site capture data points into electronic forms that submit data directly into the database. This means that the task of data entry shifts from the data capturer to clinical study staff. While this sounds incredibly efficient, it should be kept in mind that requiring clinical teams to enter data means that they have to be trained in data entry and have to allow time in their schedules for data entry and data query resolution.

DATABASE DESIGN AND BUILD

Structure/Design

Good database design starts with a proper understanding of the variables, data types, and data structure required to perform the analyses proposed in the protocol. When designing eCRFs, pay attention to logical flow of items, the need for instructional text, programmed edit checks, skipping patterns, etc. (see Fig. 10.2). The overall design of the database should be documented with grids or diagrams specifying the relationships between data tables and elements.

Useful Tips: Notes on Database Design

- *Logical flow of items*:
    Make sure that the items follow on each other as naturally as possible in the database, and following the questions on paper forms as closely as possible.
- *Instructional text*:
    Include instructions in the database to guide the capturer, for example, by giving details of where to locate certain information in the paper forms.
- *Programmed edit checks*:
    One can set up the database to perform checks on each field as it is entered, and alert the capturer to possible errors. For example, if there is a field in the database collecting weight in kilograms, it can be set up to flag the field if the capturer enters an improbable value like "305"; the capturer can then correct the value before saving it into the database.
- *Skipping patterns*:
    Sometimes there are items that depend on previous items, and one can set up the eCRFs to automatically skip/hide items that are not applicable, which prevents errors and makes the data entry process smoother. For example, there may be an item recording the sex of a patient, and a subsequent item that asks whether the patient is currently pregnant; the subsequent items only need to be completed if the answer to the first item was "female."

Software Selection

Clinical studies increasingly make use of specialized software systems developed specifically for research data. These systems make it easier to comply

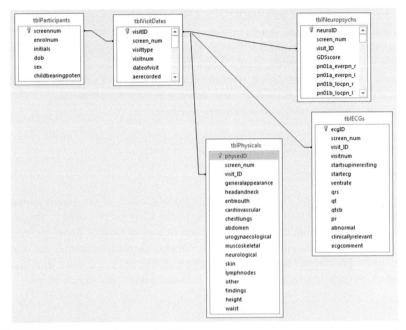

FIGURE 10.2   Example diagram of database structure.

with regulations and to connect eCRFs to the underlying database, and usually come with built-in features like visit-scheduling, audit trails, and data
resolution workflows. Some systems even combine the processes of defining
data fields for data tables and designing eCRFs. Some systems are only able
to capture data as long as there is a stable Internet connection at the site of
capture, while others may be able to collect data "offline." Certain systems
can handle importing of existing or third-party data better than others. While
some systems may include limited data summary abilities (e.g., how many
males and females enrolled or how many participants completed study),
others do not and will require the data to be exported in order to compile
even basic summaries. Of course, there are commercially priced and free/
open source systems to choose from as well. It is highly advisable to get the
input from site staff as well as data management when selecting a particular
software system.

Building/Development

The actual tables, variables, data types, allowable values, and indexes
("links" between data elements) have to be created one by one. The resulting
structure of the database should be documented with variable types, response
options, and details of relationships between data tables (Fig. 10.2). Codes
used in the database should be documented and stored securely (Fig. 10.3).

Item name (variable name)	Label (displayed on screen)	Section label	Response options (or allowable range/values)	Data type	Tested value	Comment
VSTM	Time	Vitals	hh:mm	String		
VSTEST_PULSE	Pulse	Vitals	50–120	Whole number		
VSTEST_SYSBP	BP-systolic	Vitals	90–140	Whole number		
VSTEST_DIABP	BP-diastolic	Vitals	60–90	Whole number		
VSTEST_OXYSAT	SpO₂	Vitals	60–100	Whole number		
VSSTAT_TEMP	Temp done	Vitals	Yes, No	String		
VSTEST_TEMP	Temp	Vitals	35.0-40.0	Decimal number		
...						

FIGURE 10.3 Database testing worksheet.

Alpha Testing

The person or group that creates the database is responsible for the first round of testing of the database, also called alpha testing. This involves testing how the database handles expected (normal) values, extreme values (very high or very low values), and erroneous values. Any special features and functions (e.g., backups) should also be tested thoroughly to ensure that they work as expected. This process uncovers any revisions that need to be made to the database and culminates in an updated database and database specification document.

Beta Testing

The database must now be tested for a second round, this time by persons *other* than those that created the database (called beta testing). This round of testing should ideally be performed by end users of the database, that is, the data capturers or clinical staff who will be entering the data, or persons who are peer representatives of those roles. Again the database should be tested on how it handles expected, extreme, and erroneous values, and how the special features and functions perform. Any errors uncovered are corrected and the database specification document updated.

User Acceptance

The Principal Investigator (PI) retains overall responsibility for the study, including the study database, and should sign off on the final database specifications. Upon acceptance, the SOPs for the use of the study database can be compiled by the database designer.

Third-Party Data

If any of the data are to be provided electronically by a third party (e.g., laboratory vendor), this should be discussed and the procedures and conditions documented up front. It is best practice to test the data transfer and import process prior to any real data collection. The PI remains responsible for the data, thus it is important to ensure that third-party data vendors are held to the same standards as the study team. Any third-party vendor should be able to supply the PI with their SOPs. If the third party does not have any, suggest that the study team partner with the vendor and draft the SOPs together—that way the PI can ensure that the third-party SOPs fit in with the study's overall data management plan and compliance requirements.

IMPLEMENT

Data Entry

Establish a SOP that fulfills the necessary compliance requirements, for data entry from paper forms (source documents/paper CRFs) into the database (or eCRFs). The data capturer performs visual checks on paper forms to ensure that data are legible, logical, and complete and signed off by the appropriate staff member before entering it into the database. Any errors or discrepancies must be raised with the staff member involved and must be corrected on the paper forms before it is entered into the database. Data entry should be tracked using a database completion log (Fig. 10.4).

Source Verification

The data that have been entered into the database must then be compared to the paper forms by someone other than the original capturer, for verification. Any errors or discrepancies must be raised with and corrected by the original capturer. Source verification should be tracked on the database completion log as well.

Participant ID		101				
Visit ☐	CRF ☐	QC on source	List of corrections:	Corrections made	Data entry	Source verification
Screen	Informed cons.	Checked ☐ initials:		Corrected ☐ initials:	Captured ☐ initials:	Verified ☐ initials:
Screen	Screening Q	Checked ☐ initials:		Corrected ☐ initials:	Captured ☐ initials:	Verified ☐ initials:
Screen	Demographics	Checked ☐ initials:		Corrected ☐ initials:	Captured ☐ initials:	Verified ☐ initials:
Screen	Med. history	Checked ☐ initials:		Corrected ☐ initials:	Captured ☐ initials:	Verified ☐ initials:
...						

FIGURE 10.4 Database completion log.

Data Resolution

After checking data against the source documents, the data undergo a second level of quality checks. The database is checked for missing, extreme, and illogical values. This is usually done by data management staff, who will then generate data queries for the data capturer to investigate. The data capturer performs at least the following steps in response to each data query:

1. Look up the value in question in the database and in the paper form.
2. Verify the value as correct or get the necessary correction made on the paper form.
3. Update the database to make the correction, or verify that the value in the database is correct as it stands.
4. Lastly, respond to the data query in writing to confirm the steps that have been taken.

Data management staff will consider the steps that have been taken and the response to the query, and if satisfied, will close the query. If necessary, the data management staff may update the query for further clarification by the data capturer, etc. Data resolution tasks are tracked using data clarification forms (or DCFs) as well as a log of all the DCFs (Fig. 10.5). When using specialized software systems for data entry, the data queries and responses may be tracked using built-in workflow functionality, in which case the log of the DCFs can be extracted/downloaded directly from the system.

Backup

The database should be backed up on each day on which data entry, source verification, or data resolution activities have taken place. Backups should be documented in a database backup log (Fig. 10.6).

Participant ID	DCF no.	DCF raised by	DCF resolved by	Corrections made to database	Filed with CRF
101	1	AS	CG	Y	Y
...					

FIGURE 10.5　Data clarification form log.

Manual backup location		G:\\StudyData\Backups	
Date	Time	Backup no.	Backup made by
25 Jan 2016	16:48	1	AS
...			

FIGURE 10.6　Database backup log.

DATABASE LOCK

Record Locking

Once a particular record has been entered, verified, and resolved, the data management staff will lock the record, which prevents it from being edited further. When using specialized software systems, this functionality may be built-in and may allow records to be locked form-by-form, or may allow an entire record to be locked at once.

Record Signing

Once records are locked, they can be signed off. Signing off a record means that the PI has verified that the record is ready for analysis. In the case of specialized software systems, this can be an electronic built-in functionality.

Data Export

Once records have been locked and signed, the data management team will export the data from the database system to a format that can be used for statistical analysis. Data export files must be treated with the same compliance requirements in mind as the database itself. Identifying information must be protected from unauthorized access at all times. Extracted data sets should also be backed up.

ANALYZE

Besides having to consider the relevant compliance requirements, another important principle to strive for during data analysis is reproducibility. That means keeping track of everything that has been done to the data, any recoding of variables, newly calculated/derived variables, transformations performed on the data, etc. Keeping track means that the analysis can be validated by external sources if necessary. It also means that the analysis can be repeated easily—for example, if a mistake in the analysis is uncovered, it can be traced back and corrected. Keep track of who has access to copies of the extracted data sets.

PUBLISH

Academic/Industry Publications

The purpose of the research is to generate knowledge and it is an ethical requirement to share the findings—this is often best achieved through publishing the results. Many journals/publications will require that the (deidentified) data set used to perform the analyses be made available along with the manuscript.

Final Report and Data Submissions to Regulators

Compile the final research report or other required submissions. Regulators/ funders may require that the (deidentified) data set used to perform the analyses be made available to the regulator/funder directly or on a particular platform along with the submission.

DATA SHARING AND ARCHIVE

After the final data have been exported and analyzed, it is time to consider data sharing and archiving. The purpose of archiving is to be able to retrieve the data again in the future. Computer storage space is no longer a problem, so it is probably not necessary to ever destroy data completely, but follow the protocol or data management plan specifications.

Curation Centers

Data curation centers accept (deidentified) data sets and perform quality checks on them. Curation centers then store the data and can make the data sets available for sharing with appropriate parties. A curation center also serves an archiving function, in that the researcher can access their own data sets again through the curation center.

Repositories

Data repositories function almost like curation centers, except that they do not usually perform quality checks, but make the data sets available for sharing with appropriate parties, and provide the researcher with access to their own data sets again in the future.

"Cloud"-Based and Local Archives

Researchers may also choose to keep their own archived data in the "cloud" or on physical computer hardware. When choosing this do-it-yourself method of archiving, it is important to have a plan in place to review the archive every 5 years or so. Computer technology changes constantly and the media on which the data sets are stored may become obsolete and unusable in just a few years' time. At each review time point, consider whether it may be necessary to transfer the data sets onto different storage media instead, or reconsider whether it may be appropriate to deposit the data sets into a repository or curation center that did not exist previously.

SUMMARY

This chapter has explained all the data management steps to follow through-out the project lifecycle to ensure data of consistently good quality that meets compliance requirements and is available for future use.

REFERENCES

[1] Clinical Data Interchange Standards Consortium, CDISC. 2011. Clinical Data Acquisition Standards Harmonization (CDASH). January 18.
[2] International Conference on Harmonization (ICH) E6. 1996. Good Clinical Practice: Consolidated Guideline. ICH.
[3] Prokscha S. Practical guide to clinical data management. Taylor & Francis Group: Miami; 2012.

Chapter 11

Investigational Medicinal Product (IMP) Management

Wynand Smythe and Nicky Kramer

Chapter Outline

An Investigational Medicinal Product (IMP) is defined as "a pharmaceutical form of an active substance or placebo being tested or used as a reference in a clinical trial, including products already with a marketing authorization but used or assembled (formulated or packaged) in a way different from the authorized form, or when used for an unauthorised indication, or when used to gain further information about the authorised form."

Other medication known as Non-Investigational Medicinal Products (NIMP) may be supplied as part of the study but is not the medication being investigated. This could include products such as support or rescue medication, diagnostic, or preventative treatment, or may form part of regular medical care. These do not fall within the definition of IMP and are therefore not subject to the same regulations.

The management of IMP is an integral and essential part of a clinical trial. Pharmacists are often the responsible clinical team members involved

A Comprehensive and Practical Guide to Clinical Trials.
DOI: http://dx.doi.org/10.1016/B978-0-12-804729-3.00011-0

103

in this; however, the principle investigator (PI) may delegate this task to other suitably qualified team members, for example, those members holding a dispensing license with the appropriate regulatory authority. Pharmacists are responsible for maintaining accountability of the IMP from start to finish ensuring that the right dose is given to the right participant at the right time. However, it is important for the entire clinical team to have an understanding of the IMP, particularly the dosage form, dose unit, and route of administration.

IMP management is largely concerned with accountability and pertains to several key processes namely sourcing, receiving, storage, randomization, blinding, dispensing, and disposal/return of the IMP.

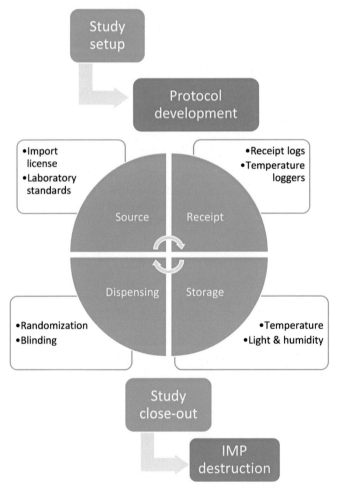

FIGURE 11.1 Flow diagram summarizing key processes in the management of IMP in clinical trials.

The study protocol should provide an overview of IMP-related activities and duties while the pharmacy manual provides details of IMP management. These details should include instructions regarding accountability processes and will dictate the processes illustrated in Fig. 11.1.

It is important to bear in mind that the rules and regulations for IMP management and pharmacy practice differ between countries and their corresponding regulatory authorities; however, the central tenet around accountability remains global and fundamental. This chapter assumes that the IMP is managed by pharmacists in a pharmacy registered with the appropriate local regulatory authorities.

WHAT TO DO IN THE PLANNING STAGES

It is important to include the pharmacy in discussions at the initial planning stages. Not all planning steps summarized below will be applicable for each study, but bear due consideration to their need.

- *Risk-assessment*

    IMP management will differ according to various factors within the study, including aspects such as the phase of study, type of IMP, and blinding requirements. As an example, if the site is required to prepare a double-blind infusion bag for an investigator-initiated study, this will present a greater risk when compared to an industry-initiated study where the sponsor provides prelabeled kits in an open-labeled study. Risk assessment is discussed in more detail under the Section "Risk-Adapted Approach to Accountability."

- *Set up agreements between relevant parties*

    Technical and contractual agreements are important to establish scope and responsibilities required by the pharmacy. Requirements could include protocol advice, attendance at site initiation visits, sourcing of IMP, standard operating procedure (SOP), and pharmacy manual development and the monitoring plan. Further discussion regarding technical agreements (TA) can be found in the Section "Technical Agreements."

    It is important to agree upfront if the sponsor will be providing the pharmacy manuals or if the site is required to develop their own. In the case of investigator-initiated research, the potential is for greater involvement of the pharmacist in providing advice and developing study-related materials such as medication labels, treatment compliance, and general accountability logs.

- *Understand sponsor requirements*

    Consider what the sponsor requires from the pharmacy in terms of facilities to manage IMP (e.g., does the IMP require refrigeration) and personnel (e.g., the need for a backup pharmacist). Requirements will vary between sponsors, so this is important to understand upfront in order to action items before the trial starts.

- *Registration and insurance documents*

  Ensure personal registration with relevant pharmacy council and indemnities are current and/or study no-fault insurance is available. Similarly, ensure the pharmacy license is current and recorded as such with the local regulatory bodies (see Chapter 4: Regulatory Requirements).

- *Training*

  Training is a continuous documented process; however, different studies may require additional study-specific training. Ensure GCP is current, and consider the need for additional training, for example, sterile technique for infusion preparations and International Air Transport Association (IATA) training for the transport of study material or IMP via airline (see Chapter 9: Training).

- *Budgeting*

  The early provision of protocols and pharmacy manuals (if available) by the sponsor to the pharmacy will assist in accurate budgeting for pharmacy services and personnel. Consider time requirements for dispensing, sourcing, shipment, and storage as well as the reconciliation and disposal costs of IMP, placebo, NIMPs, and any additional materials. Furthermore, ensure that the budget includes costs for purchasing (if required) of scales, fridges, freezers, air conditioners, etc., as well as the calibration of such equipment. Lastly, ensure that adequate time has been budgeted for trials requiring management of web-based accountability logs.

- *Checklist*

  The use of a checklist will ensure that all appropriate, important documents have been provided and are included in a master file. Refer to Table 11.1 for the "Prestudy Checklist for IMP Documentation" in the Section "Prestudy IMP Checklist."

Some Useful Tips

- When sourcing fridges for the pharmacy, in some circumstances, it may be useful to source a single large fridge rather than two smaller fridges. Alternatively, if funding is available, having extra fridges allows for backup in the event of fridge failure.
- Where possible, try have at least two pharmacists available for each study as this ensures continuity in the event of both planned (e.g., annual leave) and unplanned (e.g., sick leave) events. Furthermore, having two pharmacists better enables the pharmacy to comply with the principles within Good Manufacturing Practice (GMP).
- The pharmacy should always try to conduct a "dummy run" with the rest of the clinical team as this exercise will quickly highlight areas for further improvement, for example, time requirements to prepare and dispense the IMP to the clinical team.

ACCOUNTABILITY

Accountability is a continuous process from the start of the study until close-out, and forms the blueprint for how the IMP was managed throughout the trial. This ability to recreate exactly what happened throughout the trial is an essential part of trial documentation.

Note that industry-initiated studies generally provide documentation to be used at all study sites, whereas investigator-initiated studies may require greater assistance in developing the accountability logs and associated pharmacy manual.

RISK-ADAPTED APPROACH TO ACCOUNTABILITY

Upon agreement of the specific roles and tasks for which the pharmacy will take responsibility, the next step is to prepare the appropriate documentation, which may consist of SOPs, pharmacy manual, worksheets, and logs. Examples of these documents are available at www.crc.uct.ac.za. A risk-based approach to accountability is a common approach, which takes into account how much is known about the IMP. The general rule is that the higher the risk, the more intricate and detailed the documentation and regulatory requirements.

When analyzing risk, important things to consider are as follows:

- Type of study, for example, Phase I studies carry a greater potential risk due to the limited safety data available in humans for the IMP compared to phase III studies where more extensive data are available regarding IMP safety in humans.
- Marketing authorization of IMP, for example, commercially available formulation or new chemical entity. Similar to above, a commercially available formulation would have been administered to a greater proportion of people compared to a new chemical entity and therefore would have longer term safety data available.
- Dosage form, for example, powder for reconstitution which may require additional manipulation or manufacturing versus tablets which are dispensed to participants as provided by the sponsor.
- Preparation of IMP, for example, sterile versus nonsterile.
- Requirement for a manufacturing activity, for example, labeling (see the Section "Regulations Governing IMP Management").
- Investigator-initiated versus industry-initiated trial or study.
- IMP to be administered to the participant on site by the clinical team or taken home by the participant to be self-administered. This can impact on the level of counseling to be provided to the participant administering IMP at home to ensure that they administer the correct dosage at the appropriate time.

- Blinding procedures, for example, open label versus single or double blind. Double blind studies require significant risk management strategies to ensure that the study team is not inadvertently unblinded, which could compromise the scientific integrity of the study.

A useful tool to assess the risk of a clinical trial with regards to IMP is the Medicines and Healthcare Products Regulatory Agency (MHRA) Guideline on "Risk-adapted Approaches to the Management of Clinical Trials of IMPs" and is available via the following web-link: https://www. gov.uk/government/uploads/system/uploads/attachment_data/file/343677/Risk-adapted_approaches_to_the_management_of_clinical_trials_of_investigational_medicinal_products.pdf.

SPECIFIC PROCESSES OF ACCOUNTABILITY

Sourcing and Receiving

1. Ensure that IMPs and NIMPs are sourced and delivered ahead of participant enrollment, so pharmacists can ensure that the IMP is "safe" to use, for example, no temperature deviations have occurred during transit. Furthermore, this approach provides time to familiarize yourself with the preparing and dispensing of IMP and is particularly useful for dummy runs (practice dispensing) with the rest of the team ensuring smooth running on dosing days.
   Formulations and importation procedures vary widely. For example:
2. An industry-initiated Phase I study could involve a new IMP formulation and may need to be imported by the sponsor from a third country, hence an import license will be required. In South Africa, the regulatory-approved study protocol serves as the import license. Formulations for dummy runs could be imported ahead of time where the import license will state the IMP as a "laboratory standard, not for human consumption."
3. An investigator-initiated Phase III study may use a locally marketed product as the IMP so the pharmacist can source it directly from wholesalers without the requirement for import procedures.
4. Best practice is to source the same batch number for use throughout the study period, where possible.
5. Sourcing of placebo may present challenges, so if a study requires placebo, it is advisable to initiate that process early on, particularly if it needs to be manufactured or manipulated.
6. Accountability records for the sourcing and receipt of IMP include, for example, delivery waybills, invoices, and receipt logs.

Storage

1. Consideration needs to be given to requirements for temperature, humidity, and light control, which will dictate storage conditions during transit and once at the site. This information is available on the Certificate of Analysis (COA), prescribing information, investigators brochure (IB), or package insert for registered medicine.
2. Appropriate storage conditions need to be maintained throughout the study period, from source to destruction/disposal.
3. During transport to the site, validated boxes may be used to ensure that appropriate temperatures are maintained, ranging from ambient to freezing temperatures. Data loggers are commonly used for continuous monitoring during transit, and a process should be in place to review the data from the logger and ensure no temperature excursions have occurred.
4. Post-IMP receipt, daily temperature monitoring of the storage area is essential. Best practice is to have two temperature monitoring systems, ensuring a backup if the primary system fails. This could include manual temperature recording and continuous monitoring via temperature recording probes or data loggers. Ensure that all recording devices are regularly checked and calibrated. Automated alarms need to be set up to ensure that any temperature deviations or power failures are immediately notified to the appropriate personnel. Pharmacists are advised to regularly check, download, and acknowledge the automated temperature data (e.g., signing the print-out).
5. A written procedure for backup storage is essential and will dictate where and how to move IMP if appropriate pharmacy environment is unable to be controlled.
6. Attempt to store each study's IMP in a unique storage area, which could be a cupboard or labeled baskets if storage is limited.
7. The sponsor may issue an extended expiry date for IMPs, which requires the relabeling of IMP with the updated expiry date. The sponsor may require IMP to be returned to extend the dates, or the site may be instructed to execute the relabeling process. If relabeling is to be done at the site, ensure that the original label is not obscured by the new one and record the procedures performed during this process.
8. Accountability records for storage of IMP may include temperature logs, calibration certificates, SOPs, COAs, and IBs.

Dispensing

1. Persons delegated on the delegation log with appropriate dispensing licenses are able to dispense IMP.

2. Important checks to help ensure correct dispensing include, for example, the protocol, dose strategy, pharmacy manual, pharmacy SOPs, randomization schedules, and IMP expiry dates.
3. IMP dispensing can include a variety of procedures, depending on the formulation and requirement for nonsterile or sterile preparation.
4. The dispensing time should be established during the dummy run, ensuring the study team is made aware of potential time delays during the preparation of IMP.
5. IMP labeling needs to comply with local regulatory requirements. For example, European regulations refer to Annex 13 requirements (Articles 26−30 of Eudralex Volume 4; EU Guidelines to Good Manufacturing Practice Medicinal Products for Human and Veterinary Use: Annex 13 Investigational Medicinal Products) available via the following web-link: http://ec.europa.eu/health/files/eudralex/vol-4/2009_06_annex13.pdf
6. Labels should be reconciled before and after dispensing, and a record of this should be available.
7. Worksheets or patient dispensing logs are used to detail procedures for IMP dispensing and include a checkbox for each step of the process. These are useful tools to ensure correct dispensing and traceability.
8. If the IMP needs to be transferred, appropriate temperature control and monitoring may be needed, in addition to documentation of the transfer procedure. If the IMP is handed over to another staff member, this handover may be documented with the use of a chain of custody log and associated temperature log if required.
9. Accountability records for dispensing include, for example, dispensing worksheets/patient dispensing logs, accountability logs, label reconciliation, prescriptions, and chain of custody log.

Randomization

1. Randomization provides a mechanism for unbiased allocation of treatments. Pharmacy is often involved in ensuring correct randomization, particularly where treatments are blinded.
2. Randomization schedules provide the treatment allocations according to the proposed randomization procedure and are usually generated by the statistician or in some cases the pharmacist. The schedule can be provided in the form of automated web system, preprinted excel worksheets, or packed into sealed treatment allocation envelopes.
3. Documents related to randomization need to be stored in a secure location, with restricted access.
4. Accountability records for randomization include, for example, randomization schedules/printouts, dispensing worksheets/patient dispensing logs, accountability logs, labels, and prescriptions.

Blinding

1. Blinding of IMP is a very important area for pharmacist input and collaboration with the team. Ensuring that the IMP allocation is concealed is integral to the conduct of a blinded study.
2. Consider the type of blinding; single versus double blind, and the need for securing an appropriate placebo, that is, same smell, look, and feel.
3. Consider if a clinical team member will be administering to the participant or whether the participant will be the end-user and whether either of those need to be blinded.
4. Strategies to blind may include opaque covers for infusion bags, matching placebo, dark/colored IV lines, covering syringes with stickers, over-encapsulation of tablets or powder, and pharmacist administration directly to the participant. For example, sodium chloride or dextrose solutions could be used as a placebo for IMP that is colorless liquid and has a similar viscosity to those. However, an IMP that has a white color would not be able to use these and would require an additional blinding step, such as a black bag covering the infusion bag.
5. Ensure when dispensing that there is no possibility of unblinding. Details to remember include taking the exact same length of time for dispensing of both active and placebo, not writing batch and expiry dates on the labels that would reveal the allocation and identical positioning of the label.
6. An unblinding procedure needs to be agreed on upfront and should be available at all hours of the day, so decide whether it is best to store unblinding information in the pharmacy, online or in a locked area accessible to the PI. Unblinding could be available in the form of code break envelopes or via an electronic system.
7. Documents related to blinding need to be stored in a secure location, with restricted access.
8. Accountability records for blinding include, for example, randomization schedules/printouts, dispensing worksheets/patient dispensing logs, accountability logs, labels, and prescriptions.

Disposal

1. At the conclusion of the study, a final inventory and reconciliation is performed.
2. IMP may either be returned to the sponsor for disposal or the site may be requested to arrange for destruction with a waste disposal company.
3. Accountability records for disposal include, for example, accountability logs, disposal/destruction logs, and waste manifestation certificates issued by the disposal company.

REGULATIONS GOVERNING IMP MANAGEMENT

All countries require staff to have a working knowledge of GCP; however, some countries give further guidance regarding clinical trials and IMP management (see below).

Regulations, legislations, and directives differ between countries. South Africa pharmacists registered with the South African Pharmacy Council (SAPC) comply with the regulations of dispensing and compounding when preparing IMP, and thus need to adhere to Good Pharmacy Practice (GPP) and GMP.

The European Union provide guidelines for clinical trials, which also incorporate GMP Guidelines, and particularly for IMP within Annex 13. GMP is an aspect of Quality Assurance (QA), which is the organizational structure, procedures, processes, and resources needed to implement quality management to ensure that IMPs are consistently produced, managed, and controlled to quality standards.

Manufacture in relation to an IMP is defined as "any process carried out in the course of making the product (including repackaging and labeling), but does not include dissolving or dispersing the product in, or diluting it or mixing it with, some other substance used as a vehicle for the purposes of administering it." This has particular impact on the need for a Qualified Person (QP) whose primary legal responsibility is to certify batches prior to use in a clinical trial or prior to release for sale and placing on the market.

GMP discusses the need for independent checks, so the recommendation is to have one operator and one checker per dispensing, and a QA/QP check subsequently.

Relevant guidelines for South Africa are available are as follows:

1. Good Pharmacy Practice: http://www.e2.co.za/emags/GPPv12010/pageflip. html.
2. Good Manufacturing Practice (GMP): http://www.mccza.com/documents/ 16b9955c4.01SAGuidetoGMPJun10v5.pdf.

Relevant guidelines for the European Union are as follows:

1. EudraLex—Volume 4 Good manufacturing practice (GMP) Guidelines ("Orange Guide"): http://ec.europa.eu/health/documents/eudralex/vol-4/ index_en.htm.
2. EU Guidelines to Good Manufacturing Practice: Annex 13 Investigational Medicinal Products: http://ec.europa.eu/health/files/ eudralex/vol-4/2009_06_annex13.pdf.
3. EU Guidelines to Good Manufacturing Practice: Annex 16 Certification by a Qualified Person and Batch Release: http://ec.europa.eu/health/files/ eudralex/vol-4/pdfs-m/v4_an16_200408_en.pdf.
4. EU Guidelines to Good Manufacturing Practice: Annex 15 Qualification and Validation: http://ec.europa.eu/health/files/eudralex/vol-4/2015-10_annex15. pdf.

5. Directive 2001/83/EC relating to medicinal products for human use: http://ec.europa.eu/health/files/eudralex/vol/dir_2001_83_consol_2012/ dir_2001_83_cons_2012_en.pdf.
6. Commission Directive 2003/94/EC laying down the principles and guidelines of good manufacturing practice in respect of medicinal products for human use and investigational medicinal products for human use: http:// ec.europa.eu/health/files/eudralex/vol-1/dir_2003_94/dir_2003_94_en.pdf
7. Qualified Person Code of Conduct: http://www.rsc.org/globalassets/09-careers/personal-professional-development/professional-scientists/qp-code-of-practice.pdf.

QUALITY ASSURANCE SYSTEMS

QA systems are essential aspects of the daily running of a clinical trial, and cover people, processes, procedures, premises, and product. Guidance for Pharmaceutical Quality Systems (PQSs) are provided for by the International Council for Harmonization (ICH) Tripartite Guideline Q10, available at: http://www.ich.org/fileadmin/Public_Web_Site/ICH_Products/Guidelines/ Quality/Q10/Step4/Q10_Guideline.pdf.

Important aspects of PQS system include study and staff documentation, including communications, records of training, agreements, SOPs and manuals, monitor reports, change procedures, and corrective action and preventive actions (CAPA).

Standard Operating Procedures

SOPs that are important for the site to have include access control, IMP receipt documents, IMP quarantine, IMP storage and safe handling, IMP temperature monitoring and procedures for temperature excursions, IMP blinding/ unblinding procedures, IMP expiry date/shelf-life relabeling, IMP preparation and dispensing, line clearance, IMP return and/or disposal, IMP reconciliation, and archiving of documentation.

It is also important to ensure that these are regularly checked and updated as required and that staff are deemed competent and trained on all SOPs and study-specific procedures.

Environmental Monitoring

QA systems incorporate environmental monitoring of the preparation and dispensing area. This is particularly pertinent for microbiological and particulate monitoring in sterile environments. Guidelines are available for limits for microbiological contamination and number of permitted particles per designated area. European guidelines are available at EudraLex—Volume 4 Good manufacturing practice (GMP) Guidelines Annex 1: http://ec.europa.eu/health/files/eudralex/

vol-4/2008_11_25_gmp-an1_en.pdf. The Pharmaceutical Inspection Convention and Pharmaceutical Inspection Co-operation Scheme (jointly referred to as PIC/S) provide guidance for monitoring of the environment and can be found at http://www.picscheme.org/. According to a baseline evaluation and the level of risk, regular monitoring may be required, and trend data can be used to analyze the need for intervention and/or amended monitoring frequency.

Technical Agreements

Technical Agreements (TA) provide a framework to ensure product quality and participant safety and exist between the contract giver (e.g., sponsor) and contract acceptor (e.g., manufacturer of IMP, which may be the site). The agreement specifies the roles and responsibilities of the various parties involved in IMP management. The TA should cover topics such as appropriate regulations to comply with, provision of services and supplies, quality systems, subcontracting, complaint handling and recalls, storage and transportation, equipment and site maintenance, approval and supply of documentation, retention sample requirements, and contact details.

PRESTUDY IMP CHECKLIST

Prior to commencing the trial, ensure that all documentation is available and approved. It is helpful to have a checklist to ensure that you have been provided with all the information. Suggested documents are detailed in Table 11.1; however, not all may be required for all studies therefore assess on a case-by-case basis.

With mention to the case study used throughout this book (see Chapter 7, Planning, Appendix 7.1, and Appendix 11.1 at the end of this chapter), we provide useful considerations with regard to IMP management when planning to conduct a typical Early Phase Trial.

Keypoints
- Ensure pharmacy is consulted at study development stages, to provide insights on IMP management.
- Accountability is crucial and needs to ensure a full audit track for all procedures and processing.
- Document all training and competencies, including retraining.
- Build quality systems into each SOP and process.
- QA systems allow for complete reconstruction of the trial medication traceability.
- Consider local regulations and requirements for GCP, GMP, and/or GPP.

TABLE 11.1 Prestudy Checklist for IMP Documentation in Clinical Trials			
Study Document(s)	Required (Yes/No)	Available (Yes/No)	Version and Date
Signed protocol and amendments (if any)			
Regulatory approval(s)			
Human Research Ethics Committee (HREC) approval			
Technical agreements, e.g., with manufacturers and/or distributors			
IMP supply agreements with manufacturers			
Pharmacy manual, product specification file* or instructions for handling IMP and NIMPs			
Prescription template			
Master randomization list			
Unblinding material			
Sample labels for IMP			
Sample case report forms (CRF) or source documents			
Certificate of analysis of IMP			
Investigators brochure or package insert for IMP			
Destruction plan			
Local site SOPs and accountability records			
Marketing authorization license of manufacturing site			
Local regulatory requirements, e.g., certified QP release statement and QP declaration for the European Union			

FURTHER READING

ICH Harmonised Tripartite Guideline for Good Clinical Practice E6(R1). Available from http://www.ich.org/fileadmin/Public_Web_Site/ICH_Products/Guidelines/Efficacy/E6/E6_R1_Guideline.pdf.

Guidance for Industry E6 Good Clinical Practice: Consolidated Guidance. Available from http://www.fda.gov/downloads/Drugs/.../Guidances/ucm073122.pdf.

Definition of Investigational Medicinal Products (IMPs) and Definition of Non Investigational Medicinal Products (NIMPs).
http://ec.europa.eu/health/files/pharmacos/docs/doc2006/07_2006/def_imp_2006_07_27_en.pdf.
References used throughout.
Clinical Trials Toolkit: Trial Supplies.
http://www.ct-toolkit.ac.uk/__data/assets/pdf_file/0008/35288/Trial-Supplies-Guide.pdf.
National Pharmacy Clinical Trials Advisory Group: Professional Guidance on Pharmacy Services for Clinical Trials. Version I, October 2013.
https://www.rpharms.com/support-pdfs/professional-guidance--n-pharmacy-services-for-clinical-trials-141013.pdf.

APPENDIX 11.1   CASE STUDY: INVESTIGATIONAL MEDICINAL PRODUCT (IMP) MANAGEMENT CONSIDERATIONS IN AN EARLY PHASE STUDIES

Case study

Brief:
   "A single center, double blind, randomized, placebo-controlled Phase I study to investigate the safety, tolerability, and pharmacokinetic profile of ascending doses of CRC001 in healthy adult male volunteers."

Synopsis:
   The study will evaluate the safety, tolerability, and pharmacokinetic properties of escalating single doses of CRC001 when administered to healthy male volunteers.
   Primary objectives:
   - to investigate the safety and tolerability of CRC001 when administered to healthy participants.
   - to describe the pharmacokinetics of CRC001 in healthy participants after single dose administration.
   Secondary objectives:
   - to characterize metabolites of CRC001 present in human plasma.
   - to determine efficacy of CRC001.
Note: This case study will be used throughout the remaining chapters (see Chapter 7, Planning, Appendix 7.1).

Study Design:
   Single center, double blind, randomized, placebo-controlled, ascending dose study.
   Study will comprise of 48 healthy male volunteers between the ages of 18 and 55 years.
   Study will comprise of up to six cohorts (eight participants in each) that will receive a single, ascending dose of CRC001 to assess its safety, tolerability, and pharmacokinetic profile. The starting dose will be 5 mg.
   The data obtained from each cohort will undergo a formal review by the Safety Review Team (SRT).

Sample Size: Up to 48 participants will be enrolled.

Study Duration: Approximately 58 days for each participant, including a screening period of up to 28 days.

IMP Management Considerations:
- Phase I study therefore new IMP formulation.
- Requires some manipulation, that is, reconstitution.
- Importing as a laboratory standard to allow for dummy run to ascertain complexity of preparation and time scale for dosing days.
- IMP needs to be withdrawn into a syringe for oral dosing and labeled therefore considered GMP as per European Union standards, and so will require QP release.

Chapter 12

Collecting, Processing, and Shipment of Blood and Urine Samples

Brenda Wright

Chapter Outline

Results from analyzed blood, urine, and/or any other laboratory samples are most often part of the primary or secondary outcome measures of a clinical trial. It is therefore important that we understand the importance of appropriate sample collections and quality laboratory technique when we process and ship samples.

1. *Appropriate blood sample collection*
    a. Ensure that you have identified the participant and matched him/her to the correct sample to be collected prior to collection. Make sure that your sample is labeled with the appropriate details without jeopardizing the participant's confidentiality.
    b. Abide by specific collection requirements as per your protocol and/ or laboratory manual. There is always a good reason why these requirements are specific. Not following these instructions will affect the viability of your sample and may deliver incorrect results.
    c. Collection tubes must always be adequately filled—no less than 90% of total volume.
    d. Under filling tubes may cause significant sample dilution.
    e. Where more than one sample is taken at the same time point, be sure that you know in which sequence the samples must be collected.
    f. Never transfer blood from one collection tube to another. This may lead to further dilution of your plasma sample.

A Comprehensive and Practical Guide to Clinical Trials.
DOI: http://dx.doi.org/10.1016/B978-0-12-804729-3.00012-2
119

g. Samples must be mixed thoroughly (but gently) to ensure adequate mixing with anticoagulants, etc.

h. Over vigorous shaking will lead to hemolysis or clotting factor activity.

i. Use a discard tube first when sample is drawn using a winged collection with variable tubing length so air is not introduced into the tubes leading to underfilling.

j. Difficult sampling may lead to partially clotted, hemolyzed, or activated samples. Always document a difficult sampling on your laboratory process and/or requisition form.

k. Samples in which blood is slow to fill the collection container, where there is a prolonged use of a tourniquet, or manipulation of the vein by the needle maybe prone to develop a clot in the sample collection tube.

l. Ensure that samples are transported to the process laboratory according to specific instructions as per protocol and/or laboratory manual. For example, samples that are centrifuged at refrigerated temperatures would normally have to be placed on ice immediately after collection. Some samples will have to be agitated immediately after collection and others will have to stand upright for a certain period of time to allow clotting.

2. *Blood components* (Fig. 12.1)
   a. Red Cells: Carries oxygen and iron.
   b. Buffy Coat: Contains white cells and dense platelets.
   c. Plasma: Consists of 90% water, dissolved proteins (including antibodies), glucose, clotting factors, mineral ions, hormones, carbon dioxide.

3. *Principles of blood separation*
   a. Blood separation is achieved by sedimentation and can be defined as the partial separation or concentration of suspended solid particles from a liquid by gravity.

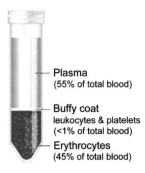

Plasma
(55% of total blood)

Buffy coat
leukocytes & platelets
(<1% of total blood)

Erythrocytes
(45% of total blood)

FIGURE 12.1   Blood components.

    b. Separation of cells are influenced not only by the gravitational force applied (centrifugation), but also the physical properties of blood, viscosity of liquid, particle density, particle size, and the fraction of dissolved solids.

    c. Differential centrifugation is used to improve the efficiency of blood component separation. During centrifugation, the accelerated force can be adjusted to separate certain cellular constituents and leave others in suspension.

4. *Centrifugation process*

There are three differential centrifugation processes used to separate whole blood into blood components:

    a. Soft or light spin: Uses low centrifugal force (slower speed) and this will produce a plasma component that contains a large fraction of platelets (platelet rich plasma) and a softly packed red cell component at the bottom of the sample tube.

    b. Hard or heavy spin: Uses high centrifugal force (faster speed and longer centrifugation time) and this produces compacted red cells at the bottom, a clear buffy coat (containing most of the white cells and platelets) with a low cellular, high volume plasma.

    c. Buffy coat spin: The buffy coat layer is located at the interface that separates the platelet-rich plasma from the packed red cells and contains less than 1% of the total volume of the blood. It contains the majority of the white blood cells as well as some of the larger more dense platelets. Blood is usually collected in a blood collection tube containing anticoagulant. Samples are collected and centrifuged at room temperature due to the vulnerability of platelets to temperature. Make sure that you follow the laboratory instructions to the point regarding centrifugation time, temperature, and resuspension.

5. *Plasma samples*

    a. Plasma is the supernatant fluid obtained when anticoagulated blood has been centrifuged.

    b. Whole blood samples are collected in containers with an anticoagulant like EDTA.

    c. The sample must be agitated gently straight after the blood is collected and should be centrifuged immediately after blood collection.

    d. If storage is necessary prior to processing, it must be done at room temperature, shielded from light and on a rocker.

    e. If the plasma is not analyzed immediately, it should be aliquoted into a 0.5 mL polypropylene tube, stored and transported at $-20°C$ or lower.

6. *Serum samples*

    a. Serum samples are blood plasma without fibrinogen or other clotting factors.

    b. Serum is clearer than plasma because of fewer proteins.

    c. Proteins are sometimes considered as interfering substances in certain tests as they react with the reagent and thereby yield inaccurate results.

    d. Whole blood samples are collected in vacutainers containing no anticoagulants.

    e. After blood is collected, samples must be rested undisturbed for ± 30 minutes at room temperature (check your laboratory instructions for exact resting time).

    f. This will allow the blood to clot.

    g. After centrifugation, it is important to immediately transfer the serum into a clean polypropylene tube.

7. Samples which are hemolyzed, lipemic, etc., can invalidate certain tests. Always annotate any abnormalities like difficult sampling, late sampling, or sample hemolyzed or lipemic on your processing log.

8. *Appropriate urine sample collection*

    a. Ensure that you have identified the participant and matched him/her to the correct sample prior to collection. Make sure that your sample is labeled with the appropriate details without jeopardizing the participant's confidentiality.

    b. Abide by specific collection requirements as per your protocol and/ or laboratory manual. There is always a good reason why these requirements are specific. Not following these instructions will affect the viability of your sample and may deliver skewed results.

    c. Store urine in the appropriate containers at the instructed temperature as described in the protocol and/or laboratory manual.

    d. Make sure that the containers are sealed properly.

9. *Appropriate storage and shipment*

    a. Blood and urine samples are stored and transported at specific temperatures.

    b. All storage facilities, that is, fridges (between 2 and 10°C) and freezers (−20 or −80°C) must have continuing temperature monitoring with available printouts of the temperatures.

    c. Ideally, manual temperatures should be taken on a daily basis as well.

    d. Equipment must be calibrated as per manufacturer's recommendation and the certificates must be filed in the Investigator Site file.

    e. Laboratory must have access to backup power in the event of a power failure.

    f. Clocks must be synchronized with the ward/consulting room clocks where samples are collected.

    g. Make sure that you have all the documentations necessary to ship the samples, for example, waybills, pro-forma invoices, etc., before your study visit.

    h. Book the courier and dry ice (if necessary) well in advance. Usually bookings are made the day before the study visit, especially if dry ice is required.

    i. If you are shipping abroad to Central Laboratories, make sure that your shipment does not arrive at the destination on a Saturday afternoon or a Sunday. Keep track of the country's public holidays as well. If you have ambient samples to ship, it is never a good idea to have your study visits on a Friday, if the destination is only reached the next day. Some ambient samples are only viable for a certain amount of hours. Check your laboratory manual and plan ahead.

    j. Make sure that the courier used is reliable and will top up with dry ice at airports when necessary.

    k. If you are aware of problems with certain couriers, inform your Sponsor and suggest couriers that are professional and efficient in your area/country.

10. All staff handling laboratory procedures and shipments must receive protocol-specific laboratory training and staff responsible for the shipment of samples to central laboratories must have relevant training. In South Africa it is called IATA training.

11. Consequences of preanalytical issues and nonadherence to protocol or laboratory manual.

    a. False positive test results maybe obtained.

    b. False negative test results maybe obtained.

    c. Incorrect titer of antibodies maybe detected.

    d. Incorrect IMP exposure (C_{max}) maybe determined.

All of the above may jeopardize any clinical trial with dire consequences, that is, incorrect results may prevent a "good drug" from further development or allow a "bad drug" to continue and maybe even get to the marketing phase.

Record all procedures to ensure an audit trail. As with all other data recorded on source documents, the laboratory procedures must be recorded as well to illustrate that the processing was done according to the prescribed protocol and/or laboratory manual.

To follow this audit trail, you need to record the whole procedure, from the time the blood was drawn, to the time it was received in the laboratory, placed into centrifuge, the time out of the centrifuge, and the time stored in the freezer.

You also need to confirm the centrifuge speed, temperature and for how long the samples were spun and at what temperature the aliquots are stored.

Do not forget to comment on the status of your sample if it is hemolyzed or lipemic, and also if it was a difficult and/or late sample.

Fig. 12.2 illustrates how all this information can be combined in one source document.

Trial site:						Protocol No.:			
Participant Intial:						Participant No.:			

Centrifuge Speed:	1500g = 3973 RPM	Time of Centrifugation:	10 min
Centrifuge Temperature:	4°C	Freezer Temperature:	−20°C
		(samples to be frozen within 30 min of plasma preparation)	

Date	Visit No.	PK Time Point	Time received in Lab	Time into Centrifuge	Time out of Centrifuge	Comment & Initial	Time into Freezer	Date Shipped	Comment & Initial
__/__/__	3	Pre-dose	_:_	_:_	_:_		_:_		
		0.5 hr post	_:_	_:_	_:_		_:_		
		1 hr post	_:_	_:_	_:_		_:_		
		2 hr post	_:_	_:_	_:_		_:_		
		3 hr post	_:_	_:_	_:_		_:_		
		4 hr post	_:_	_:_	_:_		_:_		
		6 hr post	_:_	_:_	_:_		_:_	__/__/__	
		8 hr post	_:_	_:_	_:_		_:_		
__/__/__		12 hr post	_:_	_:_	_:_		_:_		
__/__/__		24 hr post	_:_	_:_	_:_		_:_		
		48 hr post	_:_	_:_	_:_		_:_		

Study number, Visit 3 Lab Processing Log Final Version 1.0 Data Recording dated:
Refers to SOP8, Version 1 dated 2 Jan 14

QC done by: _____   Date: _____

Page 1 of 1

FIGURE 12.2 Laboratory PK process log.

Keypoints

- Appropriate sample collections and quality laboratory techniques are vital to ensure quality data, as results from the analysis of blood/urine/tissue samples are most often part of the Primary or Secondary outcome measures of a trial.
- Always follow the instructions of collection and processing as prescribed in the study protocol and/or laboratory manual.
- Staff must have protocol-specific laboratory and shipment training prior to all clinical trials.
- Annotate any abnormalities like difficult sampling, late sampling, or sample hemolyzed or lipemic on your processing log.
- Be aware of the consequences of nonadherence.
- Appropriate storage and shipment guidelines must be followed.

FURTHER READING

www.medscape.com/viewarticle/758469_4 [accessed 10.01.16].

Chapter 13

Source Document

Brenda Wright

Chapter Outline

The planning stage of a clinical trial as discussed in Chapter 7, Planning, includes the design of source documents. In this chapter we discuss the fundamental elements of quality data, definition of source data and source documents, Good Clinical Practice (GCP) requirements, responsibility, design of source documents, and version control. Practical examples are illustrated in Chapter 14, Screening, Treatment, and Safety Follow-up Visit.

1. *Source Data* are all information in original records and certified copies of original records of clinical findings, observations, or other activities in a clinical trial necessary for the reconstruction and evaluation of a trial. Source Data are contained in Source Documents (original records or certified copies).

   a. *Fundamental Elements of Quality Data:*
   The term *ALCOA* is widely used to describe these elements.

   A—Attributable: Data, findings, observations, and related documents are marked with appropriate identifiers (e.g., patient number, protocol number, sample ID) and the trial member responsible for making the entry must initial/sign and date the entry.

   L—Legible: Data should be clear and handwriting should be easy to read. This also refers to the quality of the printed documents. Electronic documents must be available in "human readable" electronic format. Text that is not legible is the same as "missing data or no documentation."

   C—Contemporaneous: Data, findings, observations, and related documents are recorded in "real time" or present time, that is, at the time they are generated and/or conducted. Any additions, deletions, or corrections to source documents should be initialed and dated the day these alterations were made. Previous data must still be legible.

A Comprehensive and Practical Guide to Clinical Trials.
DOI: http://dx.doi.org/10.1016/B978-0-12-804729-3.00013-4
© 2017 Elsevier Inc. All rights reserved.

O—Original: Data, findings, observations, and related documents are recorded for the first time. Copies of data printed on light sensitive paper like ECG printouts are made and stamped "certified a true copy." This document is then initialed and dated by the staff member making the copy.

A—Accurate: Data, findings, observations, and related documents are correct and complete. Accurate data achieve study objectives and ensure that others can replicate the results. Data should be captured consistently.

2. *Source Documents* are original documents, data, and records, and may include hospital records, participant files, laboratory reports, participant diaries, evaluation checklists, pharmacy dispensing records, photographic negatives, X-rays, ECG printouts, recorded data from automated instruments, etc.: that is, all written and printed documents that are relevant to a participant's exposure to the Investigator product, other treatments, progress of the disease course, and response to therapy.

   a. *Good quality source documents will have the following attributes:*
      i. Complete, accurate, and follow a logical sequence of events. Paints a complete picture of what happened.
      ii. Source documents are consistent, that is, all source documents match each other and tell the same story. Data entered onto source documents should not be repeated.
      iii. Source documents are locked away safely to avoid damage and/or destruction.
      iv. Determine the impact an event has elsewhere (e.g., if an Adverse Event is reported, what concomitant medications if any were taken and is it part of the participant's medical history).
      v. Source data support entries in the Case Report Forms (CRFs).
      vi. Source documents are always available, and are easy to read and understand.

3. *The Principles of ICH-GCP Regarding Source Documents*:
   i. All clinical trial information should be recorded, handled, and stored in a way that allows its accurate reporting, interpretation, and verification.
   ii. Confidentiality of records that could identify subjects should be protected.
   iii. The Investigator should ensure the accuracy, completeness, legibility, and timelines of data reported.
   iv. Data reported on CRFs that are derived from source documents should be consistent with the source documents or the discrepancies should be explained.
   v. Any change or correction should be dated, initialed, and explained (if necessary) and should not obscure the original entry (i.e., an audit trail should be maintained).

vi. Investigator/Site should maintain trial documents as specified in Essential Documents for the Conduct of a Clinical Trial and as required by the applicable regulatory requirements.

vii. Documents should be retained until at least 2 years after the last approval of a marketing application in an ICH region and until there are no pending or contemplated marketing applications or at least 2 years have elapsed since the formal discontinuation of clinical development of the Investigational Product.

viii. It is the responsibility of the Sponsor to notify the Investigator/Site as to when these documents no longer need to be retained.

ix. The Sponsor is responsible for securing agreement from all involved parties to ensure direct access to source data/documents for the purpose of monitoring and auditing by the sponsor, and inspection by domestic and foreign regulatory authorities.

x. Quality control should be applied to each stage of data handling to ensure that all data are reliable and have been processed correctly.

4. *Responsibility of the Investigator Regarding Source Documents*:

   i. The Investigator should ensure that all staff are adequately trained on the source documentation to be used for his/her trial.

   ii. Ensure the accuracy, completeness, legibility, and timelines of data reported in the CRFs.

   iii. Provide access to source documents for all clinical trial-related monitoring, audits, Institutional Review Board (IRB) review.

   iv. Ensure that quality management systems are in place for all project-related documents and procedures.

5. *Responsibility of the Study Monitor Regarding Source Data*:

   The purposes of trial monitoring are to verify that the reported trial data are accurate, complete, and verifiable from source documents, that is, checking the accuracy and completeness of the CRF entries, source documents, and other trial-related records against each other.

6. *Source Document Design*:

   Now that we know all the rules and regulations to source data we can look at the design of source documents. Source documents are your way of telling the story of the clinical trial according to the trial-specific protocol. We also have to keep in mind that we need to record enough information and in such a way that when an outside entity, such as a monitor or auditor, reviews the information, it is clearly documented what happened and when and who documented the information. This also helps when data queries come up at the end of the trial when you can no longer remember what happened at the beginning.

   Clear, concise source documents ensure accurate data entered into the database, and will definitely cut out a lot of data queries. Check your CRF or a hardcopy of your e-CRF to ensure that the information to be entered into the database is clearly documented in your source documents and that you use the same terminology as required in the CRF/e-CRF. Remember that the staff member capturing the data into the database may not necessarily have a medical background and some terms will be foreign to them.

Source documents are necessary for the reconstruction, evaluation, and validation of study related data.

They substantiate the integrity of study data, confirm observations that are recorded, and confirm the existence of participants.

Source documents confirm that safety parameters were followed per protocol.

The following information must be present in the source documents to verify that protocol requirements and safety parameters have been met. Monitors, auditors, and inspectors will look for each of these elements to be present during their reviews:

i. The informed consent process must be documented (see Chapter 14, Screening, Treatment, and Safety Follow-up Visit, Fig. 14.1).

ii. Each inclusion/exclusion criteria must be addressed and documented separately. Eligibility criteria cannot include a blanket statement (see Chapter 14, Screening, Treatment, and Safety Follow-up Visit, Fig. 14.5).

iii. Source documents supporting eligibility criteria must be filed in participant file, for example, Pathology reports, Radiographic evidence of disease, Local Laboratory reports, Medical/Surgical history, ECG printouts, etc.

iv. Clinical study required tests and procedures must be completed and recorded per protocol and "if not … why not?" Always have space at the end of your source documents where clinical notes and other incidents can be recorded (see Chapter 14, Screening, Treatment, and Safety Follow-up Visit, Fig. 14.3).

v. Participants completed, withdrawn and/or lost to follow-up must be documented.

vi. Adverse Events/Serious Adverse Events must be properly documented/reported. The process and documentation of Serious Adverse Event reporting is usually dictated by the study protocol and sponsor company in pharmaceutical trials. In Investigator trials, there should be a Standard Operating Procedure describing the process and documents required.

If you look at the examples of source documents illustrated in Chapter 14, Screening, Treatment, and Safety Follow-up Visit, you will notice that there is specific information at the top (headers included) and the bottom (footers) of these documents.

At the top of the document, you will have the name of your business, the protocol number, and the name of the document (e.g., Screening Visit,

Inclusion/Exclusion criteria, etc.). You will also always have the Participant Initials, the Participant Number, and the Visit Date. This way it is very clear who you are, which protocol you are working from, which event you are reporting, who the participant is, and when it happened. You could also display the page number in the top right-hand corner if you prefer.

At the bottom of the document, you will have the File Name (version control included), the reference to your Standard Operating Procedure and the page number of your document, preferably page ___ of ___ so that the reviewer can identify how many pages this document consist of.

7. *What is Version Control?*

It is also known as Revision Control System and is a repository of files, with monitored access and forms part of document control.

   a. Why do we need Version Control?

   It enables us to track changes made and it identifies the latest version to be used.

   b. How do we implement Version Control?

   i. Version control is always shown in the footer of your document and can be part of your File Name. (See example of source documents in Chapter 14: Screening, Treatment, and Safety Follow-up Visit.)

   ii. It starts with the first draft: Draft Version 0.1 and the date.

   iii. This draft will be sent for review. It is very important that source documents are reviewed by as many of your study team members as possible, especially the Investigator and coordinator if they are not designing the source documents themselves.

   iv. Once reviewed, changes are then made into Draft Version 0.2 with the date of changes made.

   v. When all the changes are final, documents are filed into Final Version 1.0 with appropriate date.

   vi. Should final Version 1.0 need changes, it will be filed into draft version 1.1, sent for review until approved to be placed into Final Version 2.0 with appropriate date.

   vii. Changes are never made in a Final Version.

   viii. A master copy (appropriately marked as master copy) of all final version source document templates must be filed in your site file. Previous versions must be marked as superseded. The latest version of the master copies will be used in your participant file.

8. *Electronic Source Documents (eSource):*

   a. Access to eSource must be protected by individual user name and password.

   b. eSource must have an auditable trail: time/date stamp for each entry.

   c. Study team must review the CRF prior to enrollment to ensure that their eSource document system captures all the data being requested.

    d. Design paper source for required protocol data not on your eSource.

    e. Know your system's limitations and address concerns prior to enrollment.

    f. Always have a backup plan for recording data on paper source if/when your system is down.

Keypoints

- ALCOA—Elements of Source Documentation.
- Always follow ICH-GCP guidelines regarding source documents.
- Ensure that source data are complete, accounted for, and follow a logical sequence of events.
- Ensure that source data support entries in CRF.
- Know your protocol so that protocol-specific events are recorded and not missed.
- Implement version control and quality management plan.
  REMEMBER: "If it is not documented, it is not done."
  When Monitors, Auditors, etc. call... MAY THE SOURCE BE WITH YOU!

FURTHER READING

Guidance for Industry, E6 Good Clinical Practice: Consolidated Guidance, April 1996 [accessed January 2016].

Chapter 14

Screening, Treatment, and Safety Follow-up Visit

Brenda Wright

Chapter Outline

SCREENING PERIOD

As soon as the Site has been initiated and the "green light" given, screening procedures may start. By now the potential participants must be recruited and prescreened. Most protocol designs allow ± 28 days for screening. Make sure that you allow enough time for all results to be available at the end of your screening period. Participant source document files must be prepared and training completed on all site staff.

A Comprehensive and Practical Guide to Clinical Trials.
DOI: http://dx.doi.org/10.1016/B978-0-12-804729-3.00014-6

1. Ensure that all staff working on the trial have been delegated their duties according to their qualifications by the Principal Investigator on the site delegation log (see Appendix 14.1) and that all training has been completed.

2. Allow enough time for the screening visit and warn your participants that this visit may take up to at least 4 hours of their time.

3. When the participants arrive, give them the Informed Consent Documents in the language of their choice and allow them enough time to read through it. Note the time they start reading the document on your source document (see Appendix 14.2).

4. Allow the participant the opportunity to take the Informed Consent document with them to discuss with family and/or friends should they wish to do so and return on another day to sign and complete the screening visit.

5. Depending on the nature of the trial and the size of your study team, you can book participants in groups. The Informed Consent discussion by the Investigator or suitably trained staff can be done in a group. Your Standard Operating Procedure must describe this process in detail. Discuss the content of the Informed Consent document with them and allow participants to ask questions. Sometimes one participant asking a question will prompt the others to ask questions as well. Other times participants will not want to ask questions in a group for personal reasons.

6. After the group discussion, each participant is seen separately for another discussion by the Investigator or suitably trained staff. Use this opportunity to assess your participant's understanding of the trial and participation. This can be done through careful questioning. If anything is unclear, take the time to explain again. Give the participant another opportunity to ask questions. Record all questions asked on your source document (Appendix 14.2) as well as the answers given to the participant.

7. Once this is done and the participant is willing to continue, all consent documents can be signed by the participant and the Investigator. Note the time of signature on your source document. This way you have recorded how long the Informed Consent process lasted (seeAppendix 14.2).

8. As soon as the Informed Consent document is signed by both parties, you can allocate a screening number and start with your protocol-specific screening procedures (Appendix 14.3).

9. Fig. 14.1 provides a flow diagram illustrating an easy sequence of events that normally works well when you screen more than one participant on the same day. This sequence can be changed to suit the study team, as long as the Informed Consent is signed prior to any study procedures performed. It is good practice to leave the invasive procedures (collecting of blood samples, etc.) until last. Should the participant not be eligible on any of the other investigations (e.g., BMI not within specifications or vital signs out of range), you can stop the Screening visit without the additional risk of performing a venipuncture. Unnecessary laboratory costs can be avoided this way as well.

10. Investigator will collate all information from the screening visit and complete the Inclusion/Exclusion source document noting if participant is

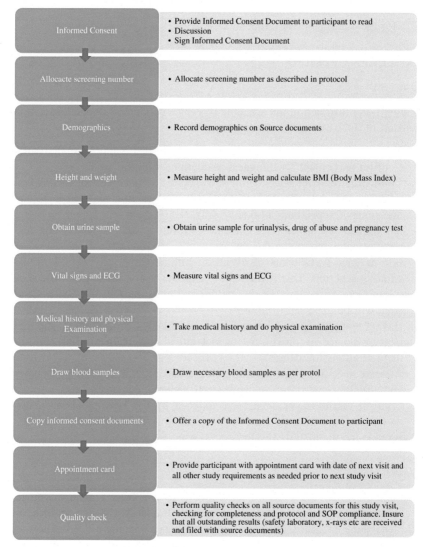

FIGURE 14.1   Sequence of events flow diagram.

eligible to be enrolled onto trial (Appendix 14.4). The Investigator must also sign and date all source documents once completed. If any information is added at a later date, the investigator must acknowledge this by initialing and dating next to or below the new information.

11. Source documents are quality checked for completeness and signed in the footer of each page (see Appendix 14.3).
12. Contact participants and discuss next visit OR explain if participant is not eligible to continue participating in the trial.
13. Prepare ward, confirm with caterers, check stock and equipment, and notify study team regarding the first admission date.

14. Check preadmission checklist to ensure everything is in place and ready for the admission day (Appendix 14.5).

TREATMENT PERIOD

Day −1

Day − 1 as illustrated in the schedule of events (Chapter 7, Appendix 7.2) is the start of the participant's treatment period.

1. Following admission, eligibility needs to be confirmed again (Appendix 14.4).
2. Confirm participant's willingness to continue with this trial.
3. Confirm participant's wellbeing and record any concomitant medication taken and/or Adverse Events (AE) reported on the applicable source documents (Appendices 14.6 and 14.7).
4. All procedures as per the schedule of events must be performed and recorded on your source documents.
5. Inform your participants of events to follow—especially Day 1 of the admission period. This is a daunting experience for participants and it is worth reassuring them the day before and ensuring that they understand what will be expected from them.
6. Have a team briefing and do a mock run of Day 1 procedures. If the dispensing doctor or pharmacist cannot attend this team briefing, inform them of admission details.
7. Allocate specific roles to team members and provide each team member with the color-coded staff schedule (see Chapter 7, Appendix 7.6).
8. Confirm that all tasks have been assigned by the Principal Investigator on the delegation log.
9. Provide the night staff with their checklists.

Day 1

1. Once all staff have reported for duty, have a brief team meeting to ensure that everybody is comfortable with the tasks assigned to them.
2. The study coordinator is normally not allocated specific tasks, but acts as back-up to the rest of the team. This way he/she can step in to assist with difficult blood sampling, etc., and avoid following time points missed.
3. Make sure all participants are wearing identification tags before dosing.
4. Perform all predose procedures.
5. Two staff members would usually perform the dosing. This could be the pharmacist and the investigator, the pharmacist and the coordinator, or the investigator and the coordinator.
6. Once the participant is identified and the IMP checked, participant is dosed according to protocol specifications. If it is an oral solution, perform a mouth check afterwards.
7. All study procedures are conducted as per protocol and recorded on Day 1 source document (Appendix 14.8).

8. Record any AE reported and concomitant medication taken during the treatment period.
9. Prior to discharge, inform your participants of their next visit date as well as study restrictions to be adhered to. Make sure that this is documented in your source document.
10. Perform quality checks on all source documents completed.
11. Ensure that data are entered timeously into the paper or electronic case report forms.
12. Perform quality checks on case report form entries as soon as possible after entry.

SAFETY FOLLOW-UP VISIT (END OF TREATMENT VISIT)

1. This is the last participant visit of your study (Appendix 14.9).
2. Confirm your participant appointments with them the day before.
3. Record all participant AE and concomitant medication taken since last visit.
4. Perform all procedures as per protocol.
5. Perform quality checks on all source documents completed.
6. Ensure that data are entered timeously into the paper or electronic case report forms.
7. Perform quality checks on case report form entries.

Keypoints

- Screening procedures may only begin when site has been initiated and the "green light" is given (all regulatory and other approvals are in place).
- Ensure that study staff have been trained and delegated their duties by the Principal Investigator and signed off on the delegation log.
- Allow enough time for the screening visit.
- Allow enough time and document the informed consent process.
- Ensure participant's eligibility prior to admission.
- Record all AE's and use of concomitant medication.
- Use preadmission checklist to ensure that everything is prepared for Day −1.
- Inform participants of events to follow.
- Allocate specific roles to team members and provide each team member with color-coded staff schedule.
- Ensure that participants wear identification tags prior to dosing.
- Observe participants for any adverse reactions postdosing.
- Confirm next visit dates with participants before discharge.
- Quality check all source documents and data entries.

FURTHER READING

Tiervlei Trial Centre, Bellville, South Africa, permission obtained May 2016.

APPENDIX 14.1   DELEGATION LOG

Trial site:		Delegation Log	
Trial No.:		Principal Investigator:	

Notes for completing this document:
- Complete legibly, name as included on CV
- Enter all dates in the DD-MMM-YY format
- Use date "Authorised from" and "Authorised to" to record staff changes during the study
- Additional tasks assigned to site staff during the trial conduct should be captured on a new line
- Initials should be as per corrections in source documents / CRF
- Complete detail on total number of pages not later than the Close-Out Visit

Full name of Site Staff	Role in Trial	Full signature	Initials	Authorised Task Numbers	From (date)	Signature of Principal Investigator	To (date)	Signature of Principal Investigator

List of duties:
1. Obtain Informed Consent: Information to participants on all aspects of the trial (e.g. purpose, investigational product, treatments, benefits, risks, trial procedures, invasive procedures, compensation, legal rights, insurance, confidentiality of data)
2. Medical Assessments and trial-related medical decisions (e.g. participant's eligibility for inclusion in the trial, physical examination, evaluation of AE, SAE, interpretation of special investigations.
3. IP: receipt of consignments, handling, storing (blinded)
4. IP: handling, dispensing, accountability (un-blinded)
5. IP: handling and administration
6. Randomization procedures (IWRS)
7. Collection, handling of blood, urine or other biological samples
8. Measuring & recording ECG, Vital signs, measuring height & weight
9. Source document completion / corrections
10. Data entry / correction into the e-CRF
11. Recruitment and scheduling appointments
12. Processing of PK samples
13. Connecting and discontinuing ECG holters
14. Quality Control and Quality Assurance

APPENDIX 14.2 INFORMED CONSENT PROCESS SOURCE DOCUMENT

Trial site:		Informed Consent Process			
Protocol No.:					
Subject Initials:		Subject No.:			
Date of informed consent:	__/__/____			Version:	
Date of informed consent: (HIV)	__/__/____			Version:	
Date of informed consent: (Parmacogenetic)	__/__/____		N/A ☐	Version:	
Date of informed consent: (Intensive PK)	__/__/____		N/A ☐	Version:	
Start Time of IC Process:	___:___	Stop Time of IC Process:	___:___		

	Yes	No
Obtain the consent of participant only after REC has approved in writing the information and consent form		
Fully inform participant before they agree to take part in the trial		
Give the participant oral and written information that is free of jargon and easy to understand		
Adequate time given to participant to read ICF in preferred language		
Answer their questions accurately and honestly		
Ensure that they understand the answers		
Ensure that neither the investigator nor staff coerce participant to take part or continue to take part in the trial		
Inform the participant in writing regarding any new information that may change their decision about taking part in the trial, after approval of REC		
Ensure that the participant and the person who informs them, signs (full names) and date the consent form, and are given copies		
Process: Give the participant enough time and opportunity to ask questions about the trial		
Questions asked (if applicable), by participant, responses given and participant's satisfaction with answers		

Consent obtained by:		**Date:**	__/__/____
Controlled by:		**Date:**	__/__/____
Notes:			
Investigator:		**Date:**	__/__/____

APPENDIX 14.3 SCREENING VISIT SOURCE DOCUMENT

Site Name:

Protocol No: **Screening Visit** (Day -28 to Day -2)

Initials: ___ ___ ___   Subject No: _____   Date: _____/_____/20____

Informed Consent signed: Y̶ / N̶

See Informed Consent Process log
Copy given to participant   Y̶ / N̶

Comment: _____

Signed: _____

General Information:

Date of Birth: _____/_____/_____

Gender: ☐ Male   ☐ Female

Home Language: ☐ English   Afrikaans
☐ Other: _____

Race: ☐ White
       ☐ Black or African American
       ☐ Asian
       ☐ American Indian or Alaska Native
       ☐ Native Hawaiian or other Pacific Islander
       ☐ Other: _____

Medical history taken:
See Medical History log

Concomitant Medication:
See Medication log

Physical examination: See Physical Exam Log

Pre-test counselling for HIV done   Y̶ / N̶

Post-test counselling for HIV done if result positive:

       Y̶ / N̶ / N/A̶

DRUG ALLERGIES: Y̶ / N̶ _____

Female patients:

Childbearing: Y̶ / N̶

If yes – Method of contraception? _____

Male patients:

Method of contraception? N/A̶ _____

Time of Height and Weight: _____h_____

☐ *Subject is wearing lightweight clothing and no shoes during weighing and measurement of height.*

Height: __ __ __.__ cm   Weight: __ __ __.__ kg

Body Mass Index: _____ kg/m²

Signed: _____

ECG: Start Rest Time: _____h_____
(see ECG print-out)

Vital Signs: Time: _____h_____

☐ Subject was in supine position at least 5 min prior to BP measurement.

BP: _____ / _____ mmHg   Heart Rate: _____ / bpm

Temperature: __ __.__

Signed: _____

Date and time of last meal and drink:
____/_____/_____   _____h____

Safety bloods drawn: Y̶ / N̶
Urine obtained for urinalysis: Y̶ / N̶
Urine for Drug of Abuse and pregnancy: Y̶ / N̶
Signed: _____

Has subject **failed** to satisfy any protocol eligibility criteria?   Y̶ / N̶

If yes: Eligibility Number : _____

Did subject terminate prior to enrolment? Y̶ / N̶

If yes: date of termination: _____/_____/_____

Primary Reason for termination:
☐ Screen Failure   ☐ Adverse Event
☐ Withdrawal of Consent
☐ Physician Decision
☐ Death   ☐ Other:
If primary reason is Withdrawal of Consent or Other specify:

Site Name:

Protocol No: **Screening Visit** (Day -28 to Day -2)

Initials: ___ ___ ___   Subject No: _____   Date: _____/_____/20____

Date of next visit: _____

Reminders:

☐ No alcohol or strenuous exercise for 48 hours prior to next visit

☐ No drug or medication to be taken unless discussed with study Investigator first

☐ Bring own toiletries and change of clothes for overnight stay

☐ No food will be allowed to be brought into the ward during the stay

NOTES:

_____   _____/_____/20____
Investigator: **Date:**

APPENDIX 14.4   ELIGIBILITY SOURCE DOCUMENT

Research Centre:		Inclusion / Exclusion Criteria				
Protocol No.:						
Subject Initials:		**Subject number:**				

INCLUSION CRITERIA					
(Each potential subject must satisfy all of the following criteria to be enrolled in the study)	Screening		Day 1		
	Yes	No	Yes	No	
1. Has completed the written informed consent process					
2. Male participants age 18 to 55 years, in good health as determined by past medical history, physical examination, vital signs, electrocardiogram, and laboratory tests at screening					
3. Haematology, clinical chemistry and urinalysis results at screening that are within the local laboratory reference range or, if outside the range, not clinically significant as judged by the investigator and confirmed and agreed upon by the medical monitor					
4. Body weight of at least 50 kg and a body mass index (BMI) within the range of 18-32 kg/m^2					
5. Good peripheral venous access					
6. An ability to communicate well with the investigator, to understand and comply with the requirements of the study					
7. Agree to stay in contact with the study site for the duration of the study, provide updated contact information as necessary, and have no current plans to move away from the study area for the duration of the study					

EXCLUSION CRITERIA					
(Any potential subject who meets any of the following criteria will be excluded from participating in the study)	Screening		Day 1		
	Yes	No	Yes	No	
1. Any acute illness upon admission to the unit on Day -1 or prior to dosing on Day 1					
2. Use of any other investigational drug within 30 days or five half-lives (whichever is longer) prior to the first dose of CRC001					
3. A history of hypersensitivity to any drugs					
4. A history of anaphylaxis or severe allergic reaction					
5. Resting vital signs (measured 5 minutes in the supine position) at either screening or baseline outside normal ranges as determined by Investigator					
6. A history of clinically significant ECG abnormalities, or ECG abnormalities at either screening or baseline not clinically significant as judged by the investigator					

Research Centre:		Inclusion / Exclusion Criteria				
Protocol No.:						
Subject Initials:		**Subject number:**				
7. History of malignancy of any organ system (other than localised basal cell carcinoma of the skin), treated or untreated, within the past five years						
8. Fertile males, defined as all males physiologically capable of conceiving offspring UNLESS the participant agrees to use condoms and ensure that his partner(s) is either not of child-bearing potential or uses a highly effective method of contraception for the entire duration of the study and for twelve weeks following the last study drug administration						
9. Smokers (use of tobacco products) in the previous 3 months. Serum cotinine level ≥25 ng/ml						
10. Use of any prescription drugs, herbal supplements, over-the-counter medication or dietary supplements (vitamins included) within four weeks prior to initial dosing						
11. Intake of grapefruit or grapefruit juice or other products containing grapefruit within 28 days of the first drug administration of the study drug						
12. Excessive intake of caffeine drinks or energy drinks within 48 hours before admission defined as more than three 250ml cups, equivalent to roughly 250mg of caffeine						
13. Donation or loss of 400 ml or more of blood within eight weeks prior to screening or dosing						
14. Plasma donation (>100ml) within 60 days prior to dosing						
15. A history of immunodeficiency diseases, including a confirmed positive HIV test result						
16. A positive Hepatitis B surface antigen (HbsAG) or Hepatitis C antibody test result						
17. A history of drug or alcohol abuse within the 12 months prior to dosing, or evidence of such abuse as indicated by the tests and laboratory assays conducted during screening and/or baseline						
18. Any clinically significant mental disorder that could limit the validity of informed consent or the volunteer's ability to comply with protocol requirements						
Investigator:			Date:	__/__/____		

APPENDIX 14.5   PREADMISSION CHECKLIST

Trial site:		Pre-admission Checklist			
Protocol No.:					
Date:	__/__/_____	Time:	___:___		
				Yes	No
Confirm admission date with participants and remind them of restrictions					
Training logs of all team members signed and filed in Site file					
Time Sheets prepared for completion					
Confirmed caterer					
Consumables checked					
Admission ward prepared					
Equipment available - calibration certificates filed					
PK tubes and aliquot tubes labelled					
Participant files prepared					
Responsible staff member signature and date:			Date:	__/__/_____	

APPENDIX 14.6 ADVERSE EVENT SOURCE DOCUMENT

Trial site:			Adverse Event		
Protocol No.:					
Screen No.:		Initials:		AE No.:	
AE Term: *(if diagnosis not known, record symptoms; one form per AE)*					
Start Date:	__/__/____		Time:	__:__	
Date:	__/__/____		Ongoing at the end of the Trial:		

Outcome:			
Recovered/Resolved		Recovered/Resolved with Sequelae	
Recovering/Resolving		Fatal	
Not Recovered/Not Resolved		Unknown	
Intensity:			
Mild		Life threatening consequences	
Moderate		Death related to AE	
Severe or medically significant but not immediately life threatening			
Relation to DAA's:			
Reasonable Possibility		No Reasonable Possibility	
Action Taken with Study Treatment:			
Drug Interrupted		Other (specify):	
Drug Withdrawn			

	Yes	No
Concomitant or additional treatment given for this AE: *(if yes complete conmed source doc)*		
Discontinued study:		
Is this a serious adverse event?		
Notes:		

Investigator:		Date:	__/__/____

APPENDIX 14.7 CONCOMITANT MEDICATION SOURCE DOCUMENT

Screen No: _ _ _ .		Participant Initials: ___ ___ ___						
Any Prescription/non-prescription/traditional meds, vitamins, herbal/dietary supplement, or vaccinations <u>from 4 weeks before screening</u> and throughout the trial								
Medic ation Name:	Start date and time (dd/mmm/yyyy) (hh:mm)	Stop date and time (dd/mmm/yyyy) (hh:mm)	Formul ation	Do se wi th un its	Frequ ency	Route of administr ation	Indicat ion(s)	Initials and date
	__/__/_ ___ ___:___ _	__/__/_ ___ ___:___ _	☐ Ta b/cap ☐ Inj ☐ Susp ☐ Liq ☐ Dr op Other: ___			☐PO ☐IM ☐SC ☐Top ☐IV ☐IN ☐PV ☐P ☐Other: ___		_____ ____ __/__ _/__
	__/__/_ ___ ___:___ _	__/__/_ ___ ___:___ _	☐ Ta b/cap ☐ Inj ☐ Susp ☐ Liq ☐ Dr op Other: ___			☐PO ☐IM ☐SC ☐Top ☐IV ☐IN ☐PV ☐P ☐Other: ___		_____ ____ __/__ _/__
	__/__/_ ___ ___:___ _	__/__/_ ___ ___:___ _	☐ Ta b/cap ☐ Inj ☐ Susp ☐ Liq ☐ Dr op Other: ___			☐PO ☐IM ☐SC ☐Top ☐IV ☐IN ☐PV ☐P ☐Other: ___		_____ ____ __/__ _/__
	__/__/_ ___ ___:___ _	__/__/_ ___ ___:___ _	☐ Ta b/cap ☐ Inj ☐ Susp ☐ Liq ☐ Dr op			☐PO ☐IM ☐SC ☐Top ☐IV ☐IN ☐PV ☐P ☐Other:		_____ ____ __/__ _/__

Medication Name:	Start date and time(dd/mmm/yyyy)(hh:mm)	Stop date and time(dd/mmm/yyyy)(hh:mm)	Formulation	Dose with units	Frequency	Route of administration	Indication(s)	Initials and date
			Other: _____ ___			_____ _____		
	__/__/_ __ ___:__ _	__/__/_ __ ___:__ _	☐ Tab/cap ☐ Inj ☐ Susp ☐ Liq ☐ Drop Other: _____ ___			☐PO ☐IM ☐SC ☐Top ☐IV ☐IN ☐PV ☐P ☐Other: _____ _____		_____ ___ _/__ _/__
	__/__/_ __ ___:__ _	__/__/_ __ ___:__ _	☐ Tab/cap ☐ Inj ☐ Susp ☐ Liq ☐ Drop Other: _____ ___			☐PO ☐IM ☐SC ☐Top ☐IV ☐IN ☐PV ☐P ☐Other: _____ _____		_____ ___ _/__ _/__
	__/__/_ __ ___:__ _	__/__/_ __ ___:__ _	☐ Tab/cap ☐ Inj ☐ Susp ☐ Liq ☐ Drop Other: _____ ___			☐PO ☐IM ☐SC ☐Top ☐IV ☐IN ☐PV ☐P ☐Other: _____ _____		_____ ___ _/__ _/__
	__/__/_ __ ___:__ _	__/__/_ __ ___:__ _	☐ Tab/cap ☐ Inj ☐ Susp ☐ Liq ☐ Drop			☐PO ☐IM ☐SC ☐Top ☐IV ☐IN ☐PV ☐P		_____ ___ _/__ _/__

			op Other: _____ __		☐Other: _____ _____	
	___/___/_ ____ _____:____ _	___/___/_ ____ _____:____ _	☐ Ta b/cap ☐ Inj ☐ Susp ☐ Liq ☐ Dr op Other: _____		☐PO ☐IM ☐SC ☐Top ☐IV ☐IN ☐PV ☐P ☐Other: _____ _____	_____ ____ _/__ _/__
	___/___/_ ____ _____:____ _	___/___/_ ____ _____:____ _	☐ Ta b/cap ☐ Inj ☐ Susp ☐ Liq ☐ Dr op Other: _____		☐PO ☐IM ☐SC ☐Top ☐IV ☐IN ☐PV ☐P ☐Other: _____ _____	_____ ____ _/__ _/__
	___/___/_ ____ _____:____ _	___/___/_ ____ _____:____ _	☐ Ta b/cap ☐ Inj ☐ Susp ☐ Liq ☐ Dr op Other: _____		☐PO ☐IM ☐SC ☐Top ☐IV ☐IN ☐PV ☐P ☐Other: _____ _____	_____ ____ _/__ _/__
	___/___/_ ____ _____:____ _	___/___/_ ____ _____:____ _	☐ Ta b/cap ☐ Inj ☐ Susp ☐ Liq ☐ Dr op Other: _____		☐PO ☐IM ☐SC ☐Top ☐IV ☐IN ☐PV ☐P ☐Other: _____ _____	_____ ____ _/__ _/__

APPENDIX 14.8 DAY 1 SOURCE DOCUMENT

Site Name: **Day 1**   Protocol Number: _____

Initials: ___ ___ ___   Participant Number: S _____   Date: _____/_____/_____

Date and time of last meal:
(Participant to be fasting before and 4 hours after dosing)

_____/_____/_____   _____h_____

Pre-Dose Concomitant Medication: Y / N
(if yes enter on Medication Log)

Pre-Dose Adverse Events: Y / N
(if yes enter on AE Log)

Physical Examination done: Y / N
(if yes enter on physical exam source)

Urinalysis sample collected: Y / N
(enter results on Urinalysis source)

Pre Dose Vital Signs:

Start Rest time: _____h_____
Subject was in supine position at least 5 min prior to BP measurement.
Time: _____h_____

BP: _____ / _____ mmHg   Pulse : _____ / bpm

Temp: _____.___ °C

Signed: _____

Participant eligible: Y / N
Review Inclusion/Exclusion criteria
Review all Laboratory Results from Day -1

Pharmacogenetic Sample: Has participant consented to
this sample?   Y / N
If yes, draw sample with PK and Safety lab samples

Randomization:

Random Number: _____ Signed: _____

Pre-Dose PK and Safety Laboratory samples

Time: _____h_____ Done by: _____

Comment: _____

PG sample taken: Y / N

Dosing: **Time:** _____h_____

Actual dose:____mg Package ID: _____

Dosed by: _____ Checked by: _____

Mouth check done by: _____

Comment: _____

0.5hr post dose Vital Signs:

Start Rest time: _____h_____
Subject was in supine position at least 5 min prior to BP measurement.
Time: _____h_____

BP: _____ / _____ mmHg   Pulse : _____ / bpm

Signed: _____

0.5hr post dose ECG

Start Rest time: _____h_____
Subject was in supine position at least 10min prior to first ECG
measurement.

See ECG printouts as source

0.5hr Post dose PK:

Time: _____h_____ Done by: _____

Comment: _____

Site Name: **Day 1**   Protocol Number: _____

Initials: ___ ___ ___   Participant Number: S _____   Date: _____/_____/_____

1hr Post dose Vital Signs:

Start Rest time: _____h____
Subject was in supine position at least 5 min prior to BP measurement.
Time: _____h_____

BP: _____ / _____ mmHg   Pulse : _____ / bpm

Signed: _____

1hr post dose ECG

Start Rest time: _____h____
Subject was in supine position at least 10min prior to first ECG measurement.

See ECG printouts as source

1hr Post dose PK:

Time: _____h_____ Done by: _____

Comment: _____

_____

2hr Post dose Vital Signs:

Start Rest time: _____h____
Subject was in supine position at least 5 min prior to BP measurement.
Time: _____h_____

BP: _____ / _____ mmHg   Pulse : _____ / bpm

Signed: _____

2hr post dose ECG

Start Rest time: _____h____
Subject was in supine position at least 10min prior to first ECG measurement.

See ECG printouts as source

2hr Post-Dose PK:

Time: _____h_____ Done by: _____

Comment: _____

3hr Post dose Vital Signs:

Start Rest time: _____h____
Subject was in supine position at least 5 min prior to BP measurement.
Time: _____h_____

BP: _____ / _____ mmHg   Pulse : _____ / bpm

Signed: _____

3hr post dose ECG

Start Rest time: _____h____
Subject was in supine position at least 10min prior to first ECG measurement.

See ECG printouts as source

3hr Post-Dose PK:

Time: _____h_____ Done by: _____

Comment: _____

4hr Post dose Vital Signs:

Start Rest time: _____h____
Subject was in supine position at least 5 min prior to BP measurement.
Time: _____h_____

BP: _____ / _____ mmHg   Pulse : _____ / bpm

Signed: _____

4hr post dose ECG

Start Rest time: _____h____
Subject was in supine position at least 10min prior to first ECG measurement.

See ECG printouts as source

4hr Post dose PK:

Time: _____h_____ Done by: _____

Comment: _____

Site Name: _____   **Day 1**   Protocol Number: _____

Initials: ___ ___ ___   Participant Number: S _____   Date: _____/_____/_____

Lunch: see meal record log

6hr Post dose Vital Signs:

Start Rest time: _____h_____
Subject was in supine position at least 5 min prior to BP measurement.
Time: _____h_____

BP: _____ / _____ mmHg   Pulse : _____ / bpm

Signed: _____

6hr post dose ECG

Start Rest time: _____h_____
Subject was in supine position at least 10min prior to first ECG measurement.

See ECG printouts as source & check holter

6hr Post dose PK:

Time: _____h_____   Done by: _____

Comment: _____

Afternoon snack: see meal record log

8hr Post dose Vital Signs:

Start Rest time: _____h_____
Subject was in supine position at least 5 min prior to BP measurement.
Time: _____h_____

BP: _____ / _____ mmHg   Pulse : _____ / bpm

Signed: _____

8hr Post dose PK:

Time: _____h_____   Done by: _____

Comment: _____

Dinner: see meal record log

12hr Post dose Vital Signs:

Start Rest time: _____h_____
Subject was in supine position at least 5 min prior to BP measurement.
Time: _____h_____

BP: _____ / _____ mmHg   Pulse : _____ / bpm

Signed: _____

12hr Post dose PK:

Time: _____h_____   Done by: _____

Comment: _____

Late night snack: see meal record log

Site Name: **Day 1**   Protocol Number: _____

Initials: ___ ___ ___   Participant Number: S _____   Date: ____ / _____ / _____

Notes:

_____   ____ / ____ /20____
Investigator: **Date**

APPENDIX 14.9   FOLLOW-UP SOURCE DOCUMENT

Site Name:

Protocol No: **Follow-up Visit**

Initials: ___ ___ ___   Subject No: _____   Date: _____/_____/20____

Adverse Event
See AE log and update if necessary: _____

Concomitant Medication:
See Medication log

Physical examination: See Physical Exam Log

ECG: Start Rest Time: _____h_____
(see ECG printout)

Vital Signs: Time: _____h_____

☒   Subject was in supine position at least 5 min prior to
BP measurement.

BP: _____ / _____ mmHg Heart Rate: _____ / bpm

Temperature: __ __.__

Signed: _____

Date and time of last meal and drink:
____/_____/_____   _____h____

Safety bloods drawn: ☒ / ☒
Urine obtained for urinalysis: ☒ / ☒
Signed: _____

NOTES:

_____   ____/____/20____
Investigator: **Date:**

Chapter 15

Quality Management

Brenda Wright

Chapter Outline

According to the principles of International Council for Harmonization-Good Clinical Practice (ICH-GCP), quality management (QM) should be applied to each stage of data handling in clinical trials to ensure that all data are reliable and have been processed correctly.

QM is an overall quality system of all the activities involved in Quality Assurance (QA) and Quality Control (QC). This includes the assignment of roles and responsibilities, the reporting of results and the resolution of issues identified during the review process. It establishes a consistent, ongoing system of evaluation with a goal of improvement.

The objectives of a Quality System in Clinical Trials are to ensure delivery of credible and reliable data as well as ensuring compliance with ethical and regulatory requirements.

A Comprehensive and Practical Guide to Clinical Trials.
DOI: http://dx.doi.org/10.1016/B978-0-12-804729-3.00015-8
© 2017 Elsevier Inc. All rights reserved.

1. *Why is QM important?*
   a. *It inspires internal monitoring by the clinical team*:

      Accurate internal monitoring will prevent excessive data queries and assure quality data and reporting structures.

      Internal monitoring will isolate the problem and identify the root cause.

      Once the internal monitoring system is proven, the whole team will buy into the system and it can become a good team-building exercise.

   b. *Specific trends can be identified early on in the conduct of trials*:

      Internal monitoring will prevent repeated errors from happening and incorrect data recorded during the rest of the trial period.

      It will also allow the clinical team to reassess roles and responsibilities and adjust to suit the specific project/protocol.

   c. *Root causes of errors can be identified*:

      It is essential that the "why" behind the errors are investigated. This is the only way to find a solution to the problem.

      It assists the clinical team in identifying ineffective systems and/or processes.

      The root of the problem is often due to inadequate training and so suitable training can be instituted.

   d. *It emphasizes the need for standardization of internal processes*:

      When internal processes are standardized, work instructions are clear and concise making compliance a lot easier.

      Inspectors, auditors, monitors, and sponsors will feel confident about the site's abilities to conduct good quality clinical trials.

   e. *It identifies opportunities for improvement*:

      Regular feedback to the team will inspire opportunities and ideas for improvement.

      The team will feel responsible and it builds confidence in their ability.

   f. *Minimizes need for rework*:

      QM could be the biggest time and money saving exercise during your trial. Nothing wastes more time than having to repeat a study visit or procedure and then reentering the data, etc.

2. *Personnel roles and responsibility*:

   This is usually defined in the Delegation log for each trial where the Principal Investigator assigns duties and responsibilities to the Clinical Team. The CROs usually supply the delegation logs for Pharmaceutical trials, but the Site can use its own as well (Investigator Lead Trials). Site staff will also have job descriptions in place.

   See example of delegation log in Appendix 15.1.

3. *Training*:

   Training consists of policies, work instructions and standard operating procedures (SOPs) (site as well as Sponsor), protocol-specific and role-specific training, GCP, and local regulatory guidelines. All training must be appropriately documented, competencies signed off and filed. See example of training log in Appendix 15.2. This log can be modified for SOP training, site- and/or protocol-specific training.

4. *Policies and Procedures*:

   Written procedures are critical to the success of a quality system. Well-defined procedures should be implemented to describe all activities. This will ensure that standardization of processes and activities will be performed consistently in the same way and at the same level of quality. Procedures can be Policies and/or SOPs. These documents are usually compiled by the Clinical Operations Manager, but can also be done by the Project Manager or the principal investigator.

5. *How to set up a Quality System?*

   When writing your Clinical Quality Management Plan (CQMP), it is important that you describe how all information and findings are documented and who is responsible. Rather add job titles to responsibilities than names to prevent you from having to review the document every time somebody leaves or a new appointment is made. This plan should meet the specific needs of your clinical research site.

   The document could be written as a Policy or an SOP.

   The following is an example of a QM system written in a Policy format for a Clinical Trial Site. It will also include all the logs, checklists, etc., to be used. This policy can be adapted for Investigator Lead trials or Investigators who conduct clinical research from their consulting rooms, etc.

NAME OF TRIAL SITE

Quality Management Plan – Policies and Procedures

Purpose:

The QM plan outlines site-specific internal measures to be used. This plan includes QC and QA measures as well as Risk Management. QC will be ongoing to identify problems and intervene with corrective actions. QA will be comprehensive and conducted on a periodic basis. This plan based on QC and QA will ensure that data are complete, accurate, and verifiable, and that clinical research participants' rights and safety are protected. The QM plan has been developed to meet international, sponsor, and institutional regulations and guidelines, including GCP.

Definitions:

QM: An overall quality system of all the activities involved in QA and QC.

QA: All those planned and systematic actions that are established to ensure that the trial is performed and the data are generated, documented, and reported in compliance with GCP and the applicable regulatory requirements.

QC: The operational techniques and activities undertaken within the QA system to verify that the requirements for quality of the trial-related activities have been fulfilled.

Scope:

This QM Plan will be applied to all clinical research conducted by the trial site.

Section I – Responsible Persons

1. *Clinical Research Director*:

    The director of the trial site is responsible for the CQMP.

2. *Clinical Operations Managers*:

    The Clinical Operations Managers have been designated by the Clinical Research Director to be responsible for the implementation and supervision of the CQMP, including written standards, training, and ongoing assessment of use, need, and validity. They will report QM findings (problems, trends, and corrective actions), as well as protocol implementation and regulatory compliance to the CRC director. Monthly assurance reports will contain protocol-specific information and an overall summary of results. Trends and root/cause analysis will be continuously assessed by the operations managers, with input from the rest of the research team. The QM Plan and CRC SOPs will continuously be reassessed, teaching reinforced, and when necessary, adapted as problems are identified. They are trained and qualified to perform these delegated tasks.

3. *Principal Investigators*:

    All Principal Investigators are responsible for the conduct and overall management of their clinical trials. They are responsible to delegate protocol-specific tasks to appropriately trained and qualified staff.

Section II – Key QC Staff

Study Coordinators, Research Nurses, pharmacists, and Data Management staff will be responsible for the day-to-day QC activities.

Section III — Key QA Staff

Project Managers and Data Managers will be responsible for QA activities at the site.

Section IV — QM Activities and Tools

1. *Quality Control:*
   The following activities and tools will be used in the QC process:
   a. 100% of Regulatory submission documents will be checked against a Regulatory checklist for completeness and compliance before the documents are submitted.
   b. CRF (Case Report Form) or a hard copy of the e-CRF (electronic Case Report Form) will be checked against the protocol to ensure that all data to be entered into the database is compliant with the trial protocol.
   c. Draft Source Documents will be reviewed and approved before placed into final version.
   d. 100% Informed Consent verification and source document verification of entry criteria will be done prior to randomization.
   e. 100% source document checks for completeness and accuracy. This includes ensuring that all Laboratory results have been received and signed off by Investigator, checking ECG printouts for completeness (e.g., have all details been entered, has investigator signed it off and marked abnormalities as "CS" (clinically significant) or "NCS" (not clinically significant)) and has all AE's been completed, and concomitant medications recorded on source documents.
   f. 100% IP (Investigational Product) accountability checks.
   g. All source data will be QC'd on the same day or at the least the following day, after a study visit. All QC'd data will be entered on a quality check log. All findings will be addressed within 2 business days of identification.
   h. All data will be captured from source documents onto paper CRF or e-CRF within 5 business days of study visit unless otherwise stipulated in the trial protocol.
   i. 100% of data entered into the paper CRF or e-CRF will be checked against the source documents to ensure accuracy and completeness. All QC'd data will be entered on a quality check log. All findings will be addressed within 1 business day of identification.
   j. Data management staff will review 100% of CRFs prior to data entry for completeness, to ensure proper dating and signing, etc.
   k. Error tracking logs will be completed by the Data Manager. This log identifies and tracks categories of CRF errors. This information will be aggregated and reported to the site staff as a whole.

2. *Quality Assurance*:
   The following activities and tools will be used in the QA process:
   a. A periodic review is done and a sample size is decided on prior to commencement of a project. Only a percentage of participant files are reviewed. (Not less than 10%.)
   b. Source data and CRF entries are reviewed for accuracy as well as protocol and GCP compliance.
   c. Quarterly verification of regulatory/essential documents is done.
   d. At the beginning of a new trial, the first two participant records as well as the CRF's are reviewed for accuracy.
   e. The research visits completed by new staff will be reviewed on a weekly basis until satisfied with their work.
   f. All findings and progress will be entered into the appropriate logs and signed off by the appropriate staff member.
   g. Monthly Activity Reports are protocol-specific summaries of QM activities that are shared with the rest of the clinical team.
   h. Site Monitoring Reports from the Monitor are utilized as a QA tool, checking for any adverse trends or problems. These reports will be shared with the rest of the clinical team.

Section V – Key Indicators

1. These indicators are part of the review process.
2. Regulatory submission documents.
3. Informed Consent forms and processes.
4. Eligibility criteria.
5. Study visits, missed visits, tests, and procedures.
6. Concomitant/prohibited medications.
7. AE/SAE identification and reporting.
8. IP administration and accountability.
9. Investigator Site Files/Essential documents.

Section VI – Review Priorities

QC and QA are ongoing activities. Monthly QA reviews will consist of 10%, at a minimum, of the clinic records, alternating existing open protocols to assure review of all active protocols over the course of the year.
   Priorities will be in the following order:

1. New Staff: 100%, and no less than 5, of all visits completed by new staff will receive a QA review until competency is determined.
2. New Protocols: The first two records for a new protocol will receive a QA review.

3. Complex Protocols: Based on recommendations of the PI and/or Clinical Operations Managers and/or Coordinators, complex or large protocols may be targeted for an early or more thorough review.
4. Identified Recurrent Problems: Any adverse trend will be reevaluated and documents will be reviewed to assess the effectiveness of the corrective action.

Section VII — Correction Processes

Once a problem has been identified by analysis of the QA or QC findings, it will be discussed with the site staff. The root cause of a recurrent problem will be identified and actions will be taken to correct the problem based on the input from the site staff. These actions may include, but are not limited to, changing a process or form, training, or reassigning a task. And adverse trend will be reevaluated to assess the effectiveness of the corrective action.

Section VIII — QM Results Reporting

Documentation of QM findings will include:

1. date of review,
2. name of reviewer,
3. Participant Identification Number,
4. items reviewed,
5. finding/results of review,
6. time period covered by review/and or study visit number.

In addition, there will be a monthly report prepared by the Data Manager, which will include both the protocol-specific and site-specific summary of QM findings for the month. When monitoring reports are received, these findings will be included in the summary report. This report will be shared with the trial staff at team meetings. Overall QA and QC findings, corrective actions, and follow-up actions will be discussed at the team meetings. The data validation process is part of the QA process and involves: self-evident data corrections, simple validation/edit checks, more source data verification (if possible), and advanced validation/edit checks. Each of these is specified in a data validation specification document. The Data Manager may generate data queries to sites as required to resolve any problems encountered in the data validation process. The Data Manager summarizes the outcome of the data validation process in a narrative report, and may report an error rate if direct source verification was done.

Section IX – Staff Training

All new staff will have a competency-based orientation using the tools and forms from the site SOP manual. A competency checklist will be completed by both the new staff and the site-designated training mentor. Separate training for protocol-specific actions, policies, and forms will be done. Training will be documented, signed, and filed in the study Regulatory binder or the staff member's training file.

Section X – Revision/Evaluation/Reporting

Analysis of the findings and activities of the year will be reported at the annual staff meeting. At this meeting, it will be determined if any changes are to be made to the CQMP.

QUALITY ASSURANCE AND QUALITY CONTROL

Quality Control

ICH-GCP 1.47 describes QC as "the operational techniques and activities undertaken within the quality assurance system to verify that the requirements for quality of the trial-related activities have been fulfilled."

- QC is the real time, day-to-day checking activities that are done to ensure that all data collected during the clinical conduct of a trial is complete, accurate, and done on time.
- It is an ongoing process and 100% of the work is checked as soon as it is done.
- Quality checks are recorded on logs (see Appendices 15.3 and 15.4) and signed off once findings are resolved.

Examples

1. Verify that the Informed Consent Process is documented and completed, that is start time and finish time of Informed Consent Process.
2. Review and document that all Inclusion/Exclusion criteria in protocol have been checked and that participant is eligible or not to be enrolled into the trial.
3. Check and confirm that the correct dose was calculated and that the IP is administered according to protocol specifications.
4. Review of Source Documents prior to data entry and CRFs after entry for accuracy.
5. Tracking of IRB/EC (regulatory documents) communication. In South Africa we do not only have to obtain the Medicine Control Council (MCC) and Ethics approvals, but also the Provincial Government approval should the trial be conducted in the Provincial Hospitals

and/or recruitment is done from the Provincial Clinics/data basis (see Appendix 15.5).

6. All errors on study documents, for example, source documents must be corrected according to accepted practices (i.e., one line through, initial and date with an explanation of correction if not evident). When errors are corrected, you have to be able to see the original entry as well.

Quality Assurance

ICH-GCP1.46 describes QA as "all those planned and systematic actions that are established to ensure that the trial is performed and the data are generated, documented, and reported in compliance with Good Clinical Practice and the applicable regulatory requirements."

1. QA is a structured process.
2. It is done retrospectively and systematic.
3. A periodic review is done and a sample size is decided on prior to commencement.
4. It identifies key processes and selects indicators to measure.
5. Aggregates and analyses the findings.
6. Documents and reports the findings.
7. Identifies corrective action.
8. Evaluate the effectiveness of a plan.

Examples

1. Only a percentage of participant files are reviewed. The total depends on the volume of participants entered (not less than 10%) Source documents are reviewed to CRFs and the protocol for accuracy.
2. Quarterly verification of regulatory/essential documents.
3. At the beginning of a new trial, review the first couple of participant records as well as the CRFs for accuracy.
4. Review the research visits completed by new staff on a weekly basis until satisfied with their work.

When planning QC and QA activities, record what will be reviewed, how much will be reviewed and when it will be reviewed (Policy and/or SOP).

Create tools before the trial that can be modified to become protocol-specific (e.g., eligibility checklists, protocol tracking tools, QC checklists).

Develop SOPs to facilitate all processes put into place.

When you find a problem, isolate it and identify a root cause.

Document Management, Record Retention, and Reporting

Documents must be version controlled, stored in a safe environment, and clear written instructions regarding retention time must be available. All incidences like AEs, SAEs, Injuries on Duties, needle stick injuries, etc., must be documented and reported to the appropriate authorities within the specified time periods.

Corrective Action and Preventive Action

When You Find a Problem, What Do You Do?

1. Attempt to isolate the problem and identify a root cause.
2. A Root Cause Analysis is the process of identifying the most basic reason for the problem, which if eliminated or corrected would prevent the problem from reoccurring.

How do you do this? Corrective action preventive action (CAPA) is the overall process of investigating, documenting, reporting, and resolving identified problems. It also implements actions to correct identified problems, nonconformities, and undesirable situations and prevent them from recurring.

A *corrective action plan* consists of:

- isolating the problem,
- identifying the root cause,
- discussing as a team,
- developing a plan of correction,
- evaluating the effectiveness of the intervention.

A *preventive action plan* consists of:

- Action taken to remove or improve a process to prevent future occurrences of a nonconformance.
- It could be implemented as a result of corrective actions or you could implement preventive actions at any time for any process or activity, if it is believed, a deviation or nonconformity may occur because of a process or activity.

A CAPA is an in-depth analysis of the root cause of a problem, its impact on the quality of the project, and a search for an action plan that will have long-term and sustainable solutions. See examples for noncompliance log and report, illustrating how the CAPA can be recorded in Appendices 15.6 and 15.7.

Quality Risk Management

This is a systematic process for the assessment, control, communication, and review of risks to the implementation, maintenance, and continuous improvement of a quality system to manage risks to GCP and protocol compliance, participant safety, and data quality in clinical research.

There are two primary principles of quality risk management:

1. The evaluation of the risk to quality should be based on scientific knowledge and linked to the safety of the patient and
2. The level of effort, correctness, and documentation of the quality risk management process should be equal to the level of risk.

How Do You Initiate a Quality Risk Management Plan?

- Define the risk question, including relevant theories identifying the potential for risk.
- Gather background information and/or data on this potential risk.
- Identify a leader and critical resources.
- Stipulate a timeline, deliverables, and level of decision making for the risk management process.

Risk Assessments

1. Risk Assessments consist of the identification of hazards and the analysis and evaluation of risks associated with exposure to those hazards.
2. There are three essential questions that can be helpful in determining risks:
   a. What might go wrong?
   b. What is the chance it will go wrong?
   c. What are the consequences if it goes wrong?

Risk Control

Includes decision making to reduce the risk to an acceptable level and/or accept the risks. Questions to ask in assisting with the decision are:

1. Is the risk above the acceptable level?
2. What can be done to reduce or eliminate the risks?
3. What is the appropriate balance among benefits, risks, and resources?
4. Are new risks introduced as a result of the identified risks being controlled?

Sometimes it may not be possible to completely eliminate some risks. If so, a strategy should be in place to assure that the quality risk has been reduced to an acceptable level. This acceptable level will vary and should be decided on a trial-by-trial basis.

See example of spreadsheet in Appendix 15.8 based on the fictitious case study from Chapter 7, Planning:

Even though this trial would be assessed as a high-risk trial, the risk can be reduced to an acceptable level because of the following factors:

- Principal Investigator and Lead Investigator are both experienced in this field.
- The facility (Site) is suitable and equipped for this trial.
- The need for suitably trained staff has been identified and can be put in place prior to start.
- The specialized equipment will be supplied by the Sponsor and relevant training will be done.
- Tight timelines and strict Inclusion/Exclusion criteria can be negotiated with the Sponsor.

Quality Roles and Responsibilities

- *Principal Investigator*—carries the ultimate responsibility for the implementation of all aspects of the clinical research. The PI must ensure that a QM Plan is implemented at the research site.
- *Study Coordinator*—performs daily and periodic QM activities and assists in the process of improvement initiatives.
- *Data Management*—conducts QC review activities of the CRF and assists in the resolution of queries. Identifies ongoing data quality issues and assist in the process of improvement initiatives.
- *Regulatory Management*—performs ongoing review of incoming and outgoing regulatory documents. Does periodic reviews of regulatory files and assists in the development of regulatory file review tools. Assists in the process of improvement initiative.
- *Pharmacy*—develops and implements a Pharmacy QM Plan. Performs pharmacy QC and QA activities ensuring safety and standards for good pharmacy practices are upheld. Assists in the process of improvement initiative.
- *Laboratory*—develops and implements a laboratory QM Plan. Performs laboratory QC and QA activities ensuring safety, security, quality, and accuracy of results. Assists in the process of improvement initiatives.
- *Independent Monitor*—oversees the process of a clinical trial. Ensures that it is conducted, recorded, and reported in accordance with the protocol, SOPs, GCP, and the applicable regulatory requirements. They are appointed by the Sponsor to verify that the Site has implemented a competent QM system, not performing these functions on the Site's behalf.

Keypoints

- According to the principles of ICH-GCP, QM should be applied to each stage of data handling in clinical trials to ensure that all data are reliable and have been processed correctly.
- QM is an overall Quality system of all the activities involved in QA and QC.

Quality Assurance	Quality Control
Periodic objective review	Ongoing and concurrent daily activities
Retrospective and systematic	Real time, ongoing day-to-day checking
General overview of trial and systems	
Ensure that data are generated	
Ensure that data are documented and reported	100% of data are checked
	Data driven (checking of data capturing)
	Can be done by nonclinician

Policies and Procedures:

Written procedures are critical to the success of a quality system. Well-defined procedures should be implemented to describe all activities. This will ensure standardization of processes and activities will be performed consistently in the same way and at the same level of quality. Procedures can be Policies and/or SOPs.

Corrective Action and Preventive Action:

CAPA is the overall process of investigating, documenting, reporting, and resolving identified problems. It also implements actions to correct identified problems, nonconformities, and undesirable situations, and prevents them from recurring.

Quality Risk Management:

This is a systematic process for the assessment, control, communication, and review of risks to the implementation, maintenance, and continuous improvement of a quality system to manage risks to GCP and protocol compliance, participant safety, and data quality in clinical research.

Quality Roles and Responsibilities:

Needs to be defined and recorded prior to project start-up.

FURTHER READING

Department of Health. Guidelines for good practice in the conduct of clinical trials with human participants in South Africa. 2nd ed Pretoria, South Africa: Department of Health; 2006.

Guidance for Industry, E6 Good Clinical Practice: Consolidated Guidance, April 1996, accessed January 2016.

APPENDIX 15.1   DELEGATION LOG

Trial site:		Delegation Log	
Trial No.:		Principal Investigator:	

Notes for completing this document:
- *Complete legibly, name as included on CV*
- *Enter all dates in the DD-MMM-YY format*
- *Use date "Authorised from" and "Authorised to" to record staff changes during the study*
- *Additional tasks assigned to site staff during the trial conduct should be captured on a new line*
- *Initials should be as per corrections in source documents / CRF*
- *Complete detail on total number of pages not later than the Close-Out Visit*

Full name of Site Staff	Role in Trial	Full signature	Initials	Authorised Task Numbers	From (date)	Signature of Principal Investigator	To (date)	Signature of Principal Investigator

List of duties:
1. *Obtain Informed Consent: Information to participants on all aspects of the trial (e.g. purpose, investigational product, treatments, benefits, risks, trial procedures, invasive procedures, compensation, legal rights, insurance, confidentiality of data)*
2. *Medical Assessments and trial-related medical decisions (e.g. participant's eligibility for inclusion in the trial, physical examination, evaluation of AE, SAE, interpretation of special investigations.*
3. *IP: receipt of consignments, handling, storing (blinded)*
4. *IP: handling, dispensing, accountability (un-blinded)*
5. *IP: handling and administration*
6. *Randomization procedures (IWRS)*
7. *Collection, handling of blood, urine or other biological samples*
8. *Measuring & recording ECG, Vital signs, measuring height & weight*
9. *Source document completion / corrections*
10. *Data entry / correction into the e-CRF*
11. *Recruitment and scheduling appointments*
12. *Processing of PK samples*
13. *Connecting and discontinuing ECG holters*
14. *Quality Control and Quality Assurance*

APPENDIX 15.2   TRAINING LOG

Trial site:		CRC 1.3 Site Training Log		
Protocol No.:		Title:		
Name:		Initials	Date	Trainer Initials

APPENDIX 15.3   QUALITY CHECK LOG

Trial site:		Source Document QC Log		
Trial No.:		Participant ID:		
Visit	Data entered (date/initials)	Pre-entry check and findings	Resolution of findings	Resolved (date/initials)

APPENDIX 15.4 CASE REPORT FORM DATA ENTRY LOG

	University of Cape Town Clinical Research Centre		eCRF Data entry tracking log	
Trial No.:		Participant ID:		
Visit	Data entered (date/initials)	Pre-entry check and findings	Resolution of findings	Resolved (date/initials)

APPENDIX 15.5 REGULATORY TRACKING LOG

Trial site:				Regulatory Tracking Log				
Trial No.:				Participant ID:				
Protocol Number	MCC submission date	Queries answered date	MCC approval date	Ethics submission date	Queries answered date	Ethics approval date	Provincial submission date	Provincial approval date

APPENDIX 15.6   NONCOMPLIANCE LOG

Trial site:		Non-Compliance Log			
Trial No:		Sponsor:			
Major:					
Non-compliance number	Summary of non-compliance:	Date sent to REC	Date received from REC	Date sent to MCC	Date received from MCC
Minor:					
Non-compliance number	Summary of non-compliance:				
Reviewed by PI at end of study		Signature		Date	

APPENDIX 15.7 NONCOMPLIANCE REPORT

Trial site:		Non-Compliance Report	
Trial No:		Sponsor:	

Participant Screen No.	Participant initials	Start date (DD-MM-YYYY) or N/A	Stop date (DD-MM-YYYY) or N/A

Details of non-compliance:	
Term (check one)	
	Informed consent not properly obtained
	Did not meet inclusion criteria or met exclusion criteria but entered in the study
	Developed withdrawal criteria during the study but not withdrawn
	Investigational product administration non-compliance
	Procedure(s) performed out of window
	Missed procedure(s)
	Unintended un-blinding
	Non-adherence to SAE/IRE reporting requirements
	Use of prohibited concomitant medication
	Non-adherence to restrictions relating to activity, diet and other exposures
	Other

Category (see definitions overleaf):		Minor:		Major:	

Root cause analysis:

Corrective and preventive action taken (check all that apply)	
	Staff reminded/trained on protocol, GCP, regulatory or SOPs
	Compilation and implementation of approved protocol amendment
	Compilation and implementation of approved and effective update of relevant SOPs
	Other:

Non-compliance reported to (date reported or intended date):							
Sponsor/ CRO		HREC		MCC		Other	

Form reviewed by	Designation	Signature	Date

Definitions:

Noncompliance: An action by assigned staff which is not in accordance with documents applicable to the trial (e.g., trial protocol, relevant SOPs, GCP, and applicable regulations). Noncompliance can be reported by staff, identified during a site monitoring visit, an internal or external audit or during an inspection. Noncompliance may include, but is not limited to one or more of the following:

- An action specifically prohibited by the protocol or relevant document.
- An additional action not specified in the protocol or relevant document.
- An omission of an action specifically stipulated in the protocol or relevant document.

Major noncompliance: Serious and/or persistent contravention of GCP and/or trial-related procedures that have an impact on participant safety, may substantially alter risks to participants, may have an effect on the integrity of the trial data, and/or the ethics of the trial (e.g., failure to perform a required safety assessment, written informed consent not appropriately obtained before initiation of trial-related procedures).

Minor noncompliance: A contravention of GCP or the protocol that does not impact participant safety, compromises the integrity of the trial data, and/or ethics of the trial (e.g., trial visit conducted outside of required timeframe, failure of participant to return trial medication). Several minor observations may collectively be considered as equal to a major noncompliance.

Root cause analysis: The investigation and identification of underlying causes of problems or events, in order to develop and implement CAPAs, to prevent recurrence of the events.

APPENDIX 15.8   RISK ASSESSMENT

Criteria	High Risk (3 pts)	Medium Risk (2 pts)	Low Risk (1 pt)
Phase I (high risk), II (medium risk) or III (low risk)	3		
PI and lead Investigator Experience			1
Medical Emergency equipment and suitably trained staff			1
Suitable facility to conduct trial			1
Strict Inclusion/Exclusion Criteria	3		
Sponsor Timelines	3		
Sample size		2	
Blinded/Randomized		2	
Duration of study visits		2	
Specialized equipment and procedures	3		
Size and expertise of staff needed to conduct trial	3		
Total score:	15	6	3

Source: Case study from chapter 7

Chapter 16

Monitoring, Close-Out Visits, and Archiving

Brenda Wright

Chapter Outline

MONITORING

According to the Guidelines for Good Clinical Practice E6(R1), monitoring is "the act of overseeing the progress of a clinical trial, and of ensuring that it is conducted, recorded, and reported in accordance with the protocol, Standard Operating Procedures (SOPs), Good Clinical Practice (GCP), and the applicable regulatory requirement(s)" (in the country where the trial will be conducted).

It is the Sponsor's responsibility to ensure that all trials are monitored according to the International Council for Harmonization-Good Clinical Practice (ICH-GCP) guidelines. The duration of monitoring will be described in the monitoring plan. Some trials will be monitored on-site before, during, and after the trial, but in exceptional circumstances the sponsor may determine that central monitoring can determine appropriate conduct of a trial in accordance with GCP. This decision should be based on the design, objectives, complexity, size, blinding, risk, and endpoints of the trial.

Purpose of Monitoring

1. A trial monitor must verify that the rights and well-being of participants are protected.
2. It is the responsibility of the monitor to assess and confirm that the data reported are accurate and complete as recorded in the original source documents.

A Comprehensive and Practical Guide to Clinical Trials.
DOI: http://dx.doi.org/10.1016/B978-0-12-804729-3.00016-X

3. The monitor will verify that the conduct of the trial is compliant with the current approved protocol/amendment, SOPs, GCP, and the local regulatory requirements.

Responsibilities of the Monitor

1. The monitor should keep a written record of all monitoring visits, significant telephone calls, and letters to the Principal Investigator.
2. The monitor should be available at any time for consultation and be able to refer incidences and queries by the clinical study team and/or reporting of Serious Adverse Events (SAE) to the appropriate study team members and regulatory authorities as described in the protocol and/or other trial documents.

Preparing for a Monitor Visit

1. The study coordinator should be available for all monitor visits and the Principal Investigator should be available to receive and give feedback regarding the trial as well as any trial-related incidents.
2. The trial monitor should be seen as part of the study team. Build up a good working relationship with your trial monitor. Do not hesitate to ask for advice and keep the communication channels open. Remember, your monitor is your direct link with the Sponsor of the trial and is appointed by the Sponsor to assist you in collecting quality data within the timeframe as stipulated by the Sponsor.
3. Your trial monitor is also vitally important during a Sponsor Audit. They will support and assist you during the Audit and ensure that all required documentation is in place and that all noncompliances are addressed and documented.
a. *Site Initiation Meeting*
   i. The Site Initiation Meeting (SIV or SIM) will be the first monitor visit to your site.
   ii. Ensure that the venue for this meeting is large enough and invite the study team to attend this meeting. Have all study supplies on display.
   iii. The purpose of this meeting is to ensure that the site has all the required materials, for example, CRFs (where applicable), investigational product supplies, consent forms, and information leaflets.
   iv. During this visit, the monitor will also discuss the protocol and all protocol-related documents in detail. Treatment codes and the procedures for breaking the code will be explained as well as the requirements concerning the retention of records and retrieval of data. Investigator Site Files containing all the Essential documents will be presented to the site.
   v. The Site Files must have an index. Check that all documents are filed according to the index. If not make sure the monitor is aware

of outstanding documents and follow up to ensure all documents are filed.

  vi. The monitor will perform a site inspection and discuss timelines.

  vii. The frequency of the following visits will be set out in the monitor plan and will depend on the sponsor's SOPs, the number of participants involved and the nature of the study. It is standard practice that the monitor will book appointments with the site at least 2 weeks in advance. These dates are flexible depending on the availability of the Investigators, the coordinator, and the monitor.

b. *The next monitor visit will normally be after the screening visits and prior to the first dosing visit.*

  i. Ensure that all participant source documents are quality checked and signed off by the Investigator.

  ii. Original signed Informed Consent documents must be filed in the Site File and a copy must be placed in the participant file.

  iii. During this visit, the monitor will confirm and verify that the Informed Consent process is done according to local Ethics requirements and SOPs and confirm that Informed Consent was obtained prior to any other protocol activity.

  iv. The monitor will confirm that source documents are available to verify the existence of the participant. The monitor will also check that the Principal Investigator has delegated tasks to appropriately trained and qualified staff by reviewing the delegation log.

c. *The monitor will continue to visit the site during the duration of the trial to verify the following*:

  i. The investigational product(s) are dispensed to eligible trial participants according to the protocol and/or pharmacy manual. The monitor should also verify that the site is managing and storing the investigational product in accordance with ICH-GCP guidelines and that records are kept of dispensing and accountability. The monitor should also verify that participant compliance/noncompliance is documented.

  ii. Entries made into the Case Report Form are accurate. The source data should also be checked for correct labeling, legibility, dating, and signatures.

  iii. SAE, Adverse Events (AE), and concomitant medication are documented and reported correctly.

d. *Close-out meeting*

  Once the trial is complete and the Database is locked, the monitor will arrange a Close-Out meeting with the Principal Investigator and study team. During this visit, the monitor will:

  i. Ensure that the Site delegation log is completed and signed off by the Principal Investigator.

  ii. Arrange the return of all study-related equipments where necessary.

iii. Confirm or arrange for the destruction or return of investigative medicinal product.

iv. Ensure that all biological samples have been shipped to the analytical laboratories or destroyed.

v. Advise when the study documents are to be archived.

vi. Provide the Principal Investigator with the final monitor report for filing in the Investigator Site file.

e. *Archiving*

According to ICH-GCP, research records must be kept for a minimum of 2 years following the approval of the last marketing application.

The EU Directive 2005/28/EC requires essential documents to be stored for at least 5 years after the completion of the Clinical Trial.

These two guidelines are different and it is up to the site to follow the applicable guidelines as per country requirement and/or as described in the protocol. Documents should be retained in conformance with the applicable regulatory requirements of the country/countries where the product is approved. It is always good practice to have a SOP describing the archiving process.

i. The archiving of trial documents should be considered during the design phase of a trial and the costs of archiving should be considered and added to the study budget.

ii. Ensure that the space is adequate for storing your trial documents.

iii. The archive facility should be secure (access restricted and controlled) and appropriate environmental controls should be in place, for example, protection from fire, flood, and unauthorized access.

iv. Ensure that you will be able to retrieve these documents when and if needed (Audits, Inspections, etc.).

v. You may use the services of a commercial archive, but the Sponsor is ultimately responsible for the quality, integrity, confidentiality, and the ability to retrieve the documents timeously when required.

vi. Keep an Index Log to record all documents that were archived and retrieved.

vii. If the documents are kept at the Investigator Site, the Sponsors should be made aware of the arrangements, and written notice should be sent to the Sponsor if the Investigator Site is no longer able to keep the documents.

viii. The Sponsor should notify Investigators in writing when trial records can be destroyed. The reason for destruction should be documented and signed by an appropriate signature.

Keypoints

1. *Monitoring*:
   a. It is the Sponsor's responsibility to ensure that all clinical trials are monitored according to the ICH-GCP guidelines.
   b. Monitoring is "the act of overseeing the progress of a clinical trial, and of ensuring that it is conducted, recorded, and reported in accordance with the protocol, Standard Operating Procedures (SOPs), Good Clinical Practice (GCP), and the applicable regulatory requirement(s)" (in the country where the trial will be conducted).
   c. The trial monitor should be seen as part of the study team. Build up a good working relationship with your trial monitor. Do not hesitate to ask for advice and keep the communication channels open. Remember, your monitor is your direct link with the Sponsor of the trial and is appointed by the Sponsor to assist you in collecting quality data within the time-frame as stipulated by the Sponsor.
2. *Close-Out Visits*:
   a. Once the trial is complete and the Database is locked, the monitor will arrange a Close-Out meeting with the Principal Investigator and the study team.
3. *Archiving*:
   a. According to them, research records must be kept for a minimum of 2 years following the approval of the last marketing application.
   b. Documents should be retained in conformance with the applicable regulatory requirements of the country/countries where the product is approved.
   c. The archive facility should be secure (access restricted and controlled) and appropriate environmental controls should be in place, for example, protection from fire, flood, and unauthorized access.
   d. Keep an Index Log to record all documents that were archived and retrieved.
   e. The Sponsor should notify Investigators in writing when trial records can be destroyed.

FURTHER READING

Guidance for Industry, E6 (R1) Good Clinical Practice: Consolidated Guidance, April 1996, accessed February 2016.

ICH-GCP Section 1.6.

http://www.ct-toolkit.ac.uk/routemap/archiving [accessed October 2016].

Chapter 17

Audits and Inspections

Brenda Wright

Chapter Outline

AUDITS

According to the International Council for Harmonization-Good Clinical Practice (ICH-GCP) Section 1.6, an Audit is a "systematic and independent examination of trial related activities and documents to determine whether the evaluated trial related activities were conducted, and the data were recorded, analysed and accurately reported according to the protocol, sponsor's SOPs, GCP, and the applicable regulatory requirements."

INSPECTIONS

ICH-GCP Section 1.6 defines an Inspection as "An act by a Competent Authority of conducting an official review of documents, facilities, records and other resources that are deemed by the competent authority to be related to the clinical trial and that may be located at the trial site, at the sponsor and/or contract research organisation's facilities or at other establishments deemed appropriate by the Regulatory Authority."

PREPARING FOR AUDITS AND INSPECTIONS

Audits and Inspections may seem daunting but if you are prepared and you have conducted your clinical trials according to ICH-GCP, protocols, and standard operating procedures (SOPs) and policies, it should be a mere formality. Your study monitor will be an important link between you and the auditor and will normally visit your site to assist you in preparing for an

A Comprehensive and Practical Guide to Clinical Trials.
DOI: http://dx.doi.org/10.1016/B978-0-12-804729-3.00017-1

audit a few weeks prior to the audit. During this time, the following documents and procedures should be reviewed:

1. Review and update site SOPs/Policies and write additional SOPs/Policies where necessary.
2. Review all essential documentation in your site files as per ICH-GCP.
3. Ensure that all staff training documentation are updated and recorded.
4. Inform staff regarding possible audits/inspections and make sure that they understand the necessary behavior during an audit as well as the level of on-site presence required during the audit.
5. Tidy up offices and files.
6. Make labeling clear and consistent using the correct terminology.
7. Prepare adequate venue/boardroom facilities.
8. Ensure confidentiality and access control.

During an audit or inspection, there will be an opening meeting between the auditors/inspectors and the Principal Investigator/Clinical Operations manager and study team. Introduce your team to them and make sure that they sign a confidentiality agreement prior to allowing them access to any documents. Ask questions if their intentions are not clear and document the discussion.

The following are helpful hints in ensuring a smooth visit:

1. Ensure that the auditor/inspector will be accompanied at all times.
2. Ensure that necessary staff is available for interviews and feedback.
3. Be clear and concise when answering questions.
4. Do not try to answer a question that you do not know the answer. Admit that you do not know and find the appropriate team member to answer the question.

At the end of the audit/inspection, an exit meeting will be held and findings and their severity will be discussed.

The format of findings is different depending on the Regulatory Body/ Auditor and which country they are from. Make sure that this is discussed at the opening meeting and that the severity of the findings and actions to be taken for each is clear. A formal report will be issued (usually within 21 days) and there will be a time limit to when you have to submit your answers.

Keypoints

Audits/Inspections:
1. An Audit is a "systematic and independent examination of trial related activities and documents to determine whether the evaluated trial related activities were conducted, and the data were recorded, analysed and accurately
(Continued)

Keypoints (Continued)

reported according to the protocol, sponsor's SOPs, GCP, and the applicable regulatory requirements."
2. An Inspection is "an act by a Competent Authority of conducting an official review of documents, facilities, records and other resources that are deemed by the competent authority to be related to the clinical trial and that may be located at the trial site, at the sponsor and/or contract research organisation's facilities or at other establishments deemed appropriate by the Regulatory Authority."
3. Your study monitor will be an important link between you and the auditor and will normally visit your site to assist you in preparing for an audit a few weeks prior to the audit.
4. During an audit or inspection, there will be an initial meeting between the auditors/inspectors and the Principal Investigator/Clinical Operations manager and study team.
5. At the end of the audit/inspection, an exit meeting will be held and findings and their severity will be discussed.

FURTHER READING

Guidance for Industry, E6 (R1) Good Clinical Practice: Consolidated Guidance, April 1996, accessed February 2016.
ICH-GCP Section 1.6.

Glossary

ACS	acute coronary syndrome
ADR	Adverse Drug Reaction
AE	adverse event
AUC	area under the plasma concentration time curve
BUN	blood urea nitrogen
CAPA	corrective actions, preventative actions
C_{max}	maximum plasma concentration
C_{min}	minimum plasma concentration
CNS	clinically not significant
CQMP	Clinical Quality Management Plan
Cr	serum creatinine
CRA	clinical research associate
CRC	clinical research coordinator
CRF	case report form (electronic/paper)
CRO	contract research organization
CS	clinically significant
CSA	clinical study agreement
CSR	clinical study report
CTA	clinical trial agreement
CVA	cerebrovascular accident
DAE	discontinuation of investigational product due to adverse event
DAR	drug or device accountability records
DCF	data clarification form
DLT	dose limiting toxicity
DNA	deoxyribonucleic acid
DSMB	Data Safety Monitoring Board
DSMP	Data Safety Monitoring Plan
EC	Ethics Committee
ECG	electrocardiogram
e-CRF	electronic case report form
EDC	electronic data capture
EMEA	European Agency for the Evaluation of Medicinal Products
FDA	Food and Drug Administration (American)
FSFD	first subject first dose
FSFV	first subject first visit
FSLV	first subject last visit
GCP	Good Clinical Practice
GLP	Good Laboratory Practices

GMP	Good Manufacturing Practices
HAQ	Health Assessment Questionnaire
IB	investigator brochure
ICF	informed consent form
ICH	International Council for Harmonization
IEC	Independent Ethics Committee
IMP	investigative medicinal product
IND	investigational new drug
IP	investigational product
IRB	Institutional Review Board
IVRS	interactive voice recognition system
IWRS	interactive web recognition system
LDH	lactate dehydrogenase
LSLV	last subject last visit
MDR	medical device reporting
MedDRA	medical dictionary for regulatory activities
mmHg	millimeters of mercury
MOS	medical outcomes study
MTD	maximum tolerated dose
NDA	New Drug Application
NSAIDs	nonsteroidal antiinflammatory drug
NSR	nonsignificant risk (usually refers to device research)
PD	pharmacodynamic
PGx	pharmacogenetic research
PI	Principal Investigator
PK	pharmacokinetic
PMA	premarket approval
PMS	postmarketing surveillance
Prn	as needed
PRO	patient reported outcomes
QA	quality assurance
QBD	quality by design
QC	quality control
QMS	quality management system
QOL	quality of life
QTcF	QT interval corrected by the Fridericia correction formula
SAE	serious adverse event
SD	standard deviation
SDV	source document verification
SEM	standard error for the mean
SEV	site evaluation meeting
SIM	site initiation meeting
SIV	site initiation visit
SOC	standard of care
SOP	standard operating procedure
SR	significant risk (usually refers to device research)
SUM	start-up-meeting (investigator's meeting)
t1/2	half-life

Tbili	total Bilirubin
TK	toxicokinetics
TTP	time to progression
WBC	white blood cells
WBDC	web-based data capture
WHO	World Health Organisation
WMA	World Medical Association

Index

Note: Page numbers followed by "*f*" and "*t*" refer to figures and tables, respectively.

Source verification, 98
South Africa, clinical trial in, 33–34
South African National Clinical Trial Registry
 (SANCTR), 34
South African Pharmacy Council (SAPC), 112
Sponsor, 4–5, 129
 requirements, 105
 sponsor/clinical department, 24
 sponsor/marketing department, 24
Staff work schedule, 61, 74–75
Standard operating procedures (SOPs), 17, 19,
 33, 87, 93, 97–98, 105, 113, 157, 175,
 178, 181–182
Start-up meeting, 88–89
State Food and Drug Administration (SFDA),
 38
Status report, 79
Stock list, 76
 for equipment and consumables, 61–62
Study
 budget, 72–73
 calendar, 69–71
 coordinator, 166

T

Technical agreements (TA), 105, 114
Therapeutic Goods Administration (TGA),
 37–38

Third-party data, 97–98
Training, 106. *See also* Planning
 external, 88–90
 ICH-GCP guidelines, 87
 internal, 87–88
 log, 169
 for QM, 157
Treatment period, 136–137
Trial budget, 60–61
Trial calendar, 60
Trial monitoring, 129
Trial-specific stock list, 61–62

U

United Kingdom, clinical trial in,
 36–37
United States, clinical trial in, 35
US Department of Health & Human Services
 (DHHS), 35
User acceptance, 97

V

Version Control, 127–132

W

Weekly updated status report, 62–63

Printed in the United States
By Bookmasters